COLOUR
Your Life

HOWARD and DOROTHY SUN

COLOUR
Your Life

■ ◆ ▲ ● ▽ ⬟ ◆ ⬠ ● ▽ ◆ ■

Discover your true

personality through the

Colour Reflection Reading

PIATKUS

© 1992 Howard and Dorothy Sun

First published in 1992 by
Judy Piatkus (Publishers) Ltd
5 Windmill Street, London W1P 1HF

**The moral right of the authors
has been asserted**

*A catalogue record for this book is
available from the British Library*

ISBN 0–7499–1149–2

Edited by Martin Noble
Illustrations and design by Paul Saunders

Set in 10½/12½ Linotron Plantin Light by
Phoenix Photosetting, Chatham
Printed and bound in Great Britain by
Mackays of Chatham PLC, Chatham, Kent

This book is dedicated to bringing more colour into your life
and to help promote health, healing and personal growth

The essences are each
  a separate glass,
Through which beings light
  is passed.
Each tinted fragment
  sparkles in the sun.
A thousand colours,
  but the light is one.

Lao Tse

CONTENTS

PREFACE

We both became aware of colour early in our lives, and for both of us this awareness was powerfully affected by our experience of nature and the vivid colours of our respective native countries. Dorothy's parents are from Cyprus and she still recalls the effects – on childhood visits – of the strong bright colours, the clear blue sky and sea, the golden rays from the radiant sun and the deep, rich red earth. It filled her with joy when she thought of the brilliant rays of the Mediterranean sun beaming down on her skin, and she longed for those sunshine days to come to England.

As for myself, I was born and brought up in Jamaica and I vividly remember the lush green, tropical foliage of the banana trees and sugar plantations. I also remember the Caribbean sea for its crystal-clear and fresh green-turquoise colour on the north coast and the exotic coloured birds that caught my eye.

As we both grew older, our experience of colour was expressed through the colours we chose to wear in our clothes and our immediate home surroundings. I found myself naturally expressing my taste for colour by wearing colourful designs in ties, shirts and trousers.

Dorothy had her own bedroom when she was twelve years old. Although she was delighted, she felt unable to move in until the colour of the walls – an ice-cold blue, which created a cold and unwelcoming feeling – were redecorated. She chose a colour from the lighter tints of orange, peach and apricot and began her first conscious experiments with colour in decoration. Within a matter of hours she had transformed an unwelcoming atmosphere into a bright and cheerful one that suited her personality and her needs.

The awareness of colour was indelibly imprinted within us and from these early experiences we realised how important it was. Although we did not fully understand the power that colour had upon us at the time, we had a strong inner sense that there was some deeper significance to it. This instinctive recognition led to our eventual involvement in Living Colour, the colour awareness and personal growth organisation we were to establish in 1984.

Our interest in complementary medicine led us to attend colour workshops in the early part of the 1980s, but we found it was not enough in itself to satisfy our growing interest in the subject. It was not until Dorothy attended a lecture on colour therapy given by the late Comtesse Dorothy du Chêne that we saw a definite and meaningful direction. The meeting between these two Dorothys had a great influence on the path we chose to take in the years to follow and marked the beginning of an exciting journey. Comtesse du Chêne then referred us to Theophilus Heliodor Gimbel, who had been involved in pioneering work on colour for many years.

To this day we recall our first meeting with Theo Gimbel. Several 'coincidences' (or synchronistic happenings) occurred which made our coming together particularly meaningful and special. One example was an uncanny connection between our names. Dorothy's maiden name, and her surname at this time, was Theophilou. The word is of Greek origin, and means 'friend or lover of God'. Theo Gimbel's Christian name is Theophilus. My own surname is Sun, a name of Chinese origin (see my Note on Sun Yat Sen, p. 181). Theo Gimbel's middle name is Heliodor, and Helios is a Greek word for Sun. Over the next three years, we were to spend a lot of time together studying and working with Theo Gimbel, querying, learning, and experimenting with ideas on colour. This period served as a wonderful foundation for the work which followed and, looking back, it was perhaps the most valuable learning experience we could have had, given the limited courses available on colour.

Living Colour

Having qualified as colour therapists in 1983, we began to practise our skills professionally, but we soon began to realise that our training was, to a certain extent, incomplete. In order to become effective colour therapists, we needed to integrate teachings on spiritual and humanistic psychology with counselling and communication skills, so that we could help our clients more effectively. This led to an intensive further three-year, part-time process of education and research into physical, emotional and mental behaviour patterns, which eventually enabled us to synthesize our understanding into a comprehensive holistic system.

Shortly after this, Dorothy became more intensely involved in teaching counselling and communication skills, and in the running of personal support teams and group-therapy courses, while I concentrated on my life-long interest in the body and personal growth and began teaching the body-consciousness course called 'The Way of the Sun'. Both these courses were designed to relate to our work with colour, and later became parts of the complete Living Colour Training Programme.

Dorothy also introduced the aesthetics of colour by becoming a colour analysis consultant. She integrated the study of the aesthetics of colour for clothes with therapy, and in 1984 she established the first officially recognised colour therapy practice in Britain.

Interest from clients produced special one-day courses which quickly evolved into a series of weekend courses, and Living Colour became a reality. The name, chosen in 1984, was taken from the title of a poem written by myself, in May 1978 in 'Golden Spring' in Jamaica.

Living Colour

Live in colour
Nature surround us
Living vibrations
Are everywhere
Voices chanting
Candles burning
Life's turning
In Living Colour
Love in Red
Laugh in Yellow
Be in Blue

Through Living Colour
Awaken to colour
Experience colour
Heal with colour
In Living Colour
Beauty's dancing
Sunset's falling
Twilight's calling
In Living Colour
We are Colour
Living Colour

(Howard Sun © 1978)

With Living Colour's formation, we began to present our work at exhibitions. We created the Colour Reflection Reading (CRR), and its significance and effectiveness as an accurate tool for self-discovery and personal awareness became more and more apparent. As the general awareness of light and colour increases and becomes more widely recognised and accepted by more and more individuals, groups and organisations, so the value of colour therapy will be increasingly appreciated and recognised as one of the medicines of the future. Living Colour exists to provide a professional consultancy, with lectures and courses that can be tailored to suit the needs of a wide range of audiences. Our aim is to bring the significance and power of colour into people's awareness, to acquaint them with its uses for self-healing and help them to make a difference in their lives.

Howard Sun
London 1991

ACKNOWLEDGEMENTS

Our deepest gratitude to Theognosia-Theophilou, Dorothy's mother, who unfailingly supported us and encouraged us to pursue our chosen path.

Our particular thanks go to the late Comtesse Dorothy du Chêne, Theo Gimbel and Gita Bellin for their spiritual teaching, love and support. Our special thanks to our clients and students who supported us and believed in us. By sharing their lives with us we were able to learn from their teaching.

Our sincere thanks to Paris Marinakis, our dear friend, whose computer expertise provided us with a workable system that saved many hours of laborious, manual work.

We are also grateful to those close friends and family who regularly enquired after us and encouraged us during the writing of this book.

In the production of the book itself, we would like to thank our publishers and their staff, in particular, Gill Cormode for her professional guidance and also Martin Noble for his editorial revision.

INTRODUCTION

Colour has power. It can stimulate or sedate, excite or calm, feel hot or cold, irritate or bring pleasure, generate feelings of passion or uplift us spiritually. Understanding colour opens a new dimension to our awareness.

Most of us recall as children, being asked the question: 'What's your favourite colour?' We sensed, even then, that we could find out a lot about a person from their particular colour preference, even if we didn't understand why. Evidently, experiencing the energy of different colours has some sort of sensory effect on us. Our language is full of expressions which use colour to represent not only sensory data, but also emotional experience. We speak of 'feeling blue', 'seeing red', 'black fears' and 'white magic'. We call a life without emotion 'colourless' and before the glowing colour of a great stained-glass window, we can encounter some of our deepest spiritual states.

Colour can transform our environment and increase our productivity. It can enhance our social life, and improve our state of health. It can be used to develop our self-awareness and make us more fully alive and more colourful human beings. We are only beginning to understand its language and the importance of its magical message.

We hope that this book will be a guide in your journey towards self-discovery and self-healing. We have based it on a powerful exercise called the **Colour Reflection Reading** (CRR), developed over many years of practical work, through which you can raise your awareness of colour, and experience the significance of colour energy as it applies to you. You can use it to make contact with your whole being (physically, emotionally, mentally and spiritually) in a completely new way; and you can learn how to balance and change your mental state and understand and monitor your emotional life. You may even sense when you are about to fall ill, and take steps to heal yourself. And since colour communicates directly with others, you can use it to express yourself in your clothes and in your surroundings in a more powerful, individual way than ever before. We suggest that you start the book by reading Chapter 1, and doing the Reading for yourself. Then read the remaining chapters, absorbing the relevant information as you go, and return to the sections you wish to work with more specifically.

We would like to add that all the names in the case histories have been changed to preserve confidentiality.

This book can change your life. We wish you personal growth, health, healing and lots of fun.

chapter 1
■ ◆ ▲ ● ▼ ● ◆

THE COLOUR
REFLECTION READING

Colour Tests

Which colour do you like best? What does that colour say about
you as a person? The use of colour preference as an indicator of
human personality is a controversial subject, because people are
different from one another. Each of us carries our own personal
characteristics and expresses ourselves differently. There are no
two people in the world who express themselves exactly the same
way.

The psychology of colour has been researched and studied by
many – Max Pfister, Max Lüscher, E. R. Jaensch, Hermann
Rorschach, to name just a few. Each produced a system of using
colour as a means to assess people's personality traits and to help us
to understand more about ourselves. Colour tests in one form or
another have been used over the years in the search for new
methods and theories of diagnosing the mentally ill. Colour is often
used in psychiatric practices to reveal complex individual mental
and emotional characteristics and to allow deeper exploration into
the secrets of the human spirit.

Colour can have a radical influence on our lives in many ways,
and one of the most important is its effect on our emotions. Used
positively, it has a profound healing quality. You may have
experienced this while looking at spring flowers, or studying a
beautiful painting. The question is, how can we take advantage of
this wonderful source of energy and use it constructively to

enhance our well-being, improve our lives and discover more about ourselves at the same time?

Probably the most well-known colour test devised was that of Dr Max Lüscher, a university professor of psychology from Lusanne, Switzerland, whose *The Lüscher Colour Test* explains how colours correspond to personality traits. His system has been adopted by many psychologists and physicians to help them gain more information about their patients, both on a psychological and physiological level. In the test a person is asked to arrange a selection of eight colours from left to right in order of preference. An interpretation is then given of the colours best liked and disliked. The colours included are: ORANGE–RED, BRIGHT YELLOW, BLUE, GREEN, DARK BLUE, VIOLET, BROWN, NATURAL GREY AND BLACK.

Lüscher's contribution to our scientific understanding of colour cannot be underestimated. But there is a serious flaw in his colour system: when we look at the colours he chose they appear dull and drab, and bear little relation to the kinds of colours that people respond to in colour therapy and healing, colours which have been shown to radiate from the human aura (see Chapter 3) and which are generated through the chakra system. This is a system of introducing colour into the body (physically, emotionally, mentally and spiritually), through specific power centres or vortices of energy. Each one of the eight colours is associated with each of the eight chakras (for more information, see Chapter 3).

Colours for healing should be seen as radiating positively and clearly. BLACK, GREY and BROWN are colours not found within the rainbow and are not included in the colour wheel. Generally these colours are not used in healing. Of course they have positive attributes if used in the right context, but overall they are considered as dense and heavy colours unsuitable for therapeutic purposes (see p. 94). The eight colours chosen in the Colour Reflection Reading are generally experienced as positive and uplifting colours, ranging from RED to MAGENTA.

Living Colour has been developing the Colour Reflection Reading since 1985 as a practical method of using colour, both to reflect the state of a person's whole being, and to help bring more awareness and thus create a better balance in people's lives. The Colour Reflection Reading has been tested with thousands of people from all walks of life and has been taught to our students of colour therapy. It has become one of the main tools in our work, and in this chapter we describe how you can use it both for yourself and your friends, using the special cut-out colour shapes at the end of the book.

The Colour Reflection process is basically a simple, straight-forward technique available to anyone. It is an easy and accessible way to monitor what is happening, and what needs to happen, in your life. Working on many levels, physical, emotional, mental and spiritual, it could be treated as a party game, but it actually reveals profound and subtle insights and if taken seriously it can be a challenging experience.

Originally this process was developed spontaneously through our therapeutic work and study of colour psychology. We had already found a definite correlation between the colours which people react to and particular traits of personality, which holds whether they react positively, negatively, or with indifference. Eight specific colours correspond with these traits: RED, ORANGE, YELLOW, GREEN, TURQUOISE, BLUE, VIOLET and MAGENTA. These are the colours included in the Complementary Colour Wheel (see below). Colour it in if you like.

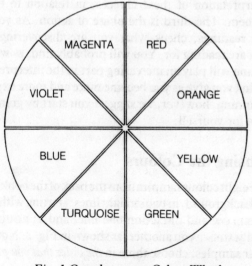

Fig. 1 Complementary Colour Wheel

We ask people to choose three colours from the colour samples and then offer an interpretation of what their choice reflects about themselves. From our experience both with our own clients and with members of the public at exhibitions, we know that this process provides an accurate reflection of peoples' emotional and physical state and needs, often at a subconscious level. The choice of certain colours can reveal emotional and physical deficiencies and imbalances, as well as powerful positive aspects of the personality of which the individual may not be aware. It can provide guidance as to how to take responsibility for overcoming problems and make the most of potential strengths. And by detecting imbalances holistically, before they are manifested at the physiological level, it can enable people to avoid illness by taking preventative action in advance. The Colour Reflection Reading can be reliably used by anyone, to give and to receive simple, accurate feedback.

The Colour Reflection Reading (CRR)

There are three steps to the reading. The first consists of making colour choices, based on personal preference. The second is the actual interpretation of these choices, in relation to the person choosing them. The third is the phase of action. As you learn to give these readings, check what you are discovering with the person you are reading for. You will probably find, as we did, that your intuition will play an increasing part in the interpretation and guidance that you give as you become more and more experienced. In the beginning, however, we suggest you start by going through the process for yourself.

1 Choosing the Colours

Cut out the eight colour samples from the back of the book. Lay them on a white background, in two straight lines, starting with RED, then ORANGE, YELLOW and GREEN on one line, and TURQUOISE, BLUE, VIOLET and MAGENTA on another, as shown in Fig. 2. Now from the eight colour samples, choose three in *the order that you prefer at this moment*.

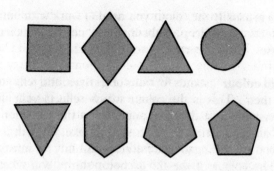

Fig. 2 How to lay out your shapes

It is important to pick your colours intuitively, without allowing mental evaluations and judgements to interfere. Take approximately 30 seconds, choose without too much thought, and forget about your favourite colours, or anything that a particular colour may remind you of, and don't try to produce a blend which harmonises together. Now place your three chosen colours separately in front of you in order of preference: first, second and third. Then put the remaining colour samples aside.

2 Interpretation

Details of the significance of each colour in each position, together with the meaning of each of the shapes, are given later in this chapter, together with examples of some actual readings. For the moment, we will focus on the meaning of the sequence itself.

The first colour represents the essence of an individual. It expresses who you really are, reflecting your basic personality, and suggests how you would normally respond to everyday situations. It is the expression of your True Self. It can also represent the predominant colour you are expressing at any given time.

The second colour speaks of the present. It relates to your current condition on all levels of the here and now: physical, emotional, mental and spiritual. This colour (or its complementary) is usually the colour you need to work with immediately and reflects your deep, subconscious needs, deficiencies, or weaknesses. It also represents your main challenge.

The third colour stands for your objectives, and tells you how to achieve them. This is the colour which reflects your innermost hopes, visions, and dreams, pointing to the direction of your destiny, and indicating the next step to take. Growth is possible here, if you are willing to take full responsibility for satisfying your needs. The colour of the third choice shows you what kind of constructive action you need to take in order to bring about a new, fresh perspective.

Colour harmonies
There are 336 possible ways of choosing from the eight colour samples. If your three choices include any two which are opposite each other on the Complementary Colour Wheel shown on page 11 this is called a 'colour harmony'. There are 144 combinations of these colours where a colour harmony can occur. Examples of colour harmonies are RED and TURQUOISE, VIOLET and YELLOW and GREEN and MAGENTA. Colour harmonies show that two colours are working exceptionally well together to bring about balance and smooth transitional phases in your life. They indicate that you are heading in the right direction, along a path that is positive and constructive and in alignment with your personality, circumstances or goals. The presence of colour harmonies means that energy is also less likely to become dispersed, dissipated or unfocused, as complementary colours act as a stabiliser and an anchor for one another. This of course reflects itself in your overall experience of life's circumstances and conditions.

Third colour harmonises with the first
Long-term developments are in alignment with your true self: success in your life's journey is indicated. This however can only occur when obstacles revealed by the second colour have been overcome.

For example, when Bill chose MAGENTA first, VIOLET second and GREEN third, he chose a colour harmony where GREEN harmonises with MAGENTA. Bill, an administrator, wants to become a community counsellor and be involved in health-care work. His future aspirations are in alignment with his basic essence and indicate a rewarding and fulfilling outcome, as long as he can overcome the challenge of VIOLET in the second position, which is to do with a lack of self-worth.

Second colour harmonises with the first

Here, the outcome of the present situation will be aligned with your true nature, assuring positive results. The uplifting and strengthening of the personality is indicated here, helping to forward the individual's growth. For example, Jane chose BLUE first, ORANGE second and YELLOW third. She chose a colour harmony where ORANGE is in alignment with BLUE. Jane, a sales representative, needed to learn how to adopt a more outgoing and positive approach to life which would help her in her work.

Third colour harmonises with the second

A favourable outcome here is also possible, although successful developments are only aligned with present conditions. The challenge of the second colour must again be overcome as a condition of achieving your final goal.

For example, Susan, a freelance graphic designer, chose BLUE first, TURQUOISE second and RED third. She chose a colour harmony where RED is aligned with TURQUOISE. Susan was currently in the process of implementing a new project which she had been working on for some time and was close to receiving some tangible results for her efforts.

When there are no colour harmonies, it does not necessarily mean that the outcome will be negative. In such cases, an especially important factor will be the predominant colour spectrum in the chosen colours, and whether they are mainly warm or cool. This gives an immediate indication of how to work towards balance. If the colours are mainly cool, then look for balance in the warm spectrum; if warm, then look for balance in the cool spectrum. This general rule can be applied to all readings. Warm colours include MAGENTA, RED, ORANGE and YELLOW. Cool colours are TURQUOISE, BLUE, and VIOLET. GREEN tends towards the cool end of the spectrum, but is often considered a neutral colour.

3 Taking Action

Now that you have completed the second step, you will be aware of some harmonies and some disharmonies in your life. It is time to take action and make practical use of your new understanding. How can you achieve this?

By acting on the information in this chapter – and in the rest of the book – you will start to integrate your personal colour(s) and this process will be both healing and empowering: by integrating your required colour(s) into your life in practical ways, you will not only come to recognise the power of colour and become more conscious of it, but the aspects of yourself that are weak or deficient will be strengthened. We will explain specific colour media and recommend how to use colour practically. There are examples and case histories to draw on, and illustrations for you to use as guidelines.

In general, we suggest you review your Colour Reflection Reading approximately once every 12 weeks as your colour balance will probably change, and the previous reading may no longer be relevant to your present situation.

The Significance of the Shapes

The eight shapes chosen for the Colour Reflection Reading and indeed all shapes generally, are derived from three basic forms – the square, the triangle and the circle.

Each shape has its own character and expresses its own energy pattern. These support the eight colours by relating to their personal qualities and overall characteristics.

Form is mostly associated with the left side of the brain, as it has to do with logic and reasoning powers. Colour on the other hand is concerned with the right side of the brain, related to feelings and sentiments, creativity and intuition. This side of the brain expresses itself through instinctive responses and an inner knowing. Colour relates more to the emotional, subconscious level and therefore helps to reveal aspects of ourselves which are not normally available to our more mechanistic, conscious side.

Together these two elements bring about complementary forces which relate to the conscious and subconscious aspects within our personality as a whole. Form predominantly relates to the conscious element within us, seeking expression in a tangible way, while colour subtly expresses the more hidden aspects of our personality. Combining these two aspects of ourselves encourages both sides of the brain to work together in a balanced and harmonious interplay.

When we choose the cards in the Colour Reflection Reading, our final choice and overall responses are based on our personal experiences and circumstances as a whole, both expressed and unexpressed. In this way the CRR helps us to discover more about ourselves, and acts as a tool for personal growth and self-development.

Colours and Their Shapes in the CRR

Red
This is represented by a square, whose straight lines suggest the most basic physical structure which reflects stability and solidity. It is the most dense colour in the spectrum and its associated shape is the most appropriate to describe groundedness, foundation, and physical strength. The square implies rigidity, tension and qualities of being held firm. These are also qualities carried by the colour RED.

Orange
This is represented by a diamond, which contains the same straight lines as RED, and in principle appears to be similar in design, except that it's been turned on its side, and, in this movement, it is stretched from above and below. It carries elements of both RED and YELLOW, the colours before and after ORANGE. The lines in ORANGE are diagonal, implying greater flexibility in movement than RED, and the emergent quality of ORANGE, shifting from the physical solidity of RED to the lightness of the next colour after ORANGE i.e. YELLOW.

Yellow

This is represented by an upright triangle. The single straight line at the base, implies a solid foundation at ground level, and the two diagonal lines meeting at the pinnacle, direct the attention upwards, as though towards the sun, and the attainment of knowledge and wisdom. This shape, like the colour, uplifts and inspires.

Green

This is represented by a circle whose shape embodies the qualities of balance and harmony and protection. It is smooth and round, with no sharp edges, reflecting the colour GREEN. It symbolises safety and freedom, a lack of imposition on others. No matter which way this shape is turned it stays the same, constant and forever neutral.

Turquoise

This is represented by a reversed triangle, implying energy focused or channelled downwards from above. The straight line is at the head of the reversed triangle, indicating that its solidity lies within the spiritual realms, while the two diagonal lines face downwards, seeking groundedness towards its complementary energy – RED. With the movement from one realm into another, many changes may be experienced, which are basic characteristics of the colour TURQUOISE.

Blue

This is represented by a hexagram which has six lines, four of which are diagonal and form two pinnacles, one at the top and one at the bottom. The pinnacle pointing upwards aspires towards spiritual wisdom and insight, while its opposite points towards the physical energy of ORANGE, BLUE's complementary colour. A further two straight lines adjoin the pinnacles on both sides, like pillars or columns, suggesting uprightness, spiritual strength and truth. The hexagram suggests gradual expansion, depth and calmness. It has the potential to act as a catalyst as the movement of energy can be focused towards either the spiritual or the physical realms.

Violet

This is represented by a reversed pentagram, this has five lines, only one of which is horizontal and this is situated at the head of the shape, implying solidity and strength within the spiritual and psychic realms. A further two lines form a pinnacle at the base of the shape, suggesting movement towards the physical dimension and the overall desire to be earthed, more stable and fixed. These are adjoined by two further diagonal lines linking the base line with the pinnacle on either side. The reversed pentagram, like VIOLET, aspires to be more practical by using its basic qualities to integrate and unify spiritual understanding with more physical and earthly expression.

Magenta

This is represented by an upright pentagram, the same shape as that of VIOLET, only in reverse. The top or head of this shape is formed by a pinnacle reflecting the desire to be further connected to the spiritual dimensions of the cosmos or universe. The base line is a straight horizontal line, indicating its ability to be stable and grounded at the same time. The pinnacle and the base are joined with two further lines, one on each side. Both of these are diagonal lines which extend upwards from the base suggesting the capacity for unfoldment. In fact the qualities related to this colour are both spiritually inclined and yet physically practical. This fits well with MAGENTA as a predominantly warm colour, which has a strong element of RED contained within it. Overall this shape symbolises wholeness, oneness and universal harmony.

The Meanings of the Colours in Each Position

The following information will form the basis of your interpretation, based on your choice of three colours.

Red

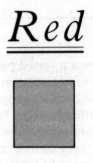

RED–FIRST POSITION

Your basic nature is to lead, rather than follow. You are an initiator, pioneer and creator, and generally you will be outgoing and assertive in life. You will also tend to be highly competitive, expressing a great deal of energy of a primal, passionate quality. RED people have an excessively strong tendency to go . . . go . . . and keep on going. Achieving, attaining, succeeding – these are your spontaneous expressions of life. You focus on a goal, and are not overly concerned with how to reach it. You do not rely on too much planning or strategy, rather on physical strength and determination. You are an active, intense and passionate individual, and your sense of physical and emotional energy is constantly heightened. It is important to learn to balance and harmonise your emotions with your logic in order to reach the level of equilibrium you seek to achieve in all aspects of your life.

RED – SECOND POSITION

Your challenge is to stimulate, energise and strengthen yourself, especially on the physical level. However, because the natural quality of RED is to externalise and constantly go forward, part of the challenge is to avoid completely exhausting and depleting your body on all levels. It is also important to be able to direct this rampant energy: patience will be a much-needed virtue for RED people. An extreme focus of RED will challenge you not to lean towards domination, aggression, confrontation, and powerful sexual stimuli. Instead, you need to work towards expressing your innate sense of love, warmth, and friendship.

RED – THIRD POSITION

Your main need is to apply yourself in some practical way. Your primary aim is to act in a down-to-earth style, both feet firmly planted on the ground. This is not a time to fantasise or delay action, but rather one of grasping opportunities that present themselves at any given moment. Deep within, you wish to act in order to establish something new and manifest it in a more tangible way. For example to move house, start a new business or to join a gym. You are ready to get up and go, though choosing RED in the third position may indicate that you are completely depleted and exhausted, especially on the physical level. Therefore, you should take 'time out' in order to calm, quieten and pacify your system. Contemplating BLUE skies, and deep BLUE or TURQUOISE seas may be an ideal replenisher.

Orange

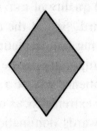

ORANGE–FIRST POSITION

You have a buoyant and ebullient nature and an enlivening, joyful, and generally excitable, happy disposition. You have a tendency to participate, enjoying life to the full, expressing courage, spontaneity and cheerfulness wherever you go. You can be talkative, not afraid to open conversations, and are outgoing and sociable. You can bring the 'kiss of life' to those with whom you interact, and uplift their spirit. However, you can often act in haste, and have a tendency to go to extremes, since you are unable to still yourself long enough to balance your normally overactive nature. This often leaves you feeling physically tired, exhausted and depleted and may lead you to be emotionally explosive. Try to balance your priorities and take stock of your wholistic situation. ORANGE people often try too hard to be *seen* to be doing the right thing. Learn to trust your basic instinctive nature.

ORANGE – SECOND POSITION

You need to become more aware of your inner being, which seeks balance, and needs to find stillness of both body and mind. Since this colour lies between YELLOW and RED, it includes both a powerfully active physical nature (RED) and a questioning (YELLOW). Such a combination of qualities gives you a drive that can often make you overpowering and overbearing to others. The challenge here is for you to adopt a more restful and relaxed attitude towards life. You need to make time for yourself, to recoup and nourish the part of you which yearns for this. Only through such periods of calm and quiet can ORANGE people move towards a more unified way of being.

ORANGE – THIRD POSITION

You need to act constructively, rather than in a destructive way. Because you have a tendency to act on the spur of the moment, little time is left for any real thought to take place. This leaves you often doubting whether your actions were the right ones. What is needed is contemplation and deliberation so that the energy can be more wisely and effectively used. You may have chosen ORANGE in the third position because you have withdrawn inwardly. Therefore the appropriate action is to step forward and be more courageous, confident, and enjoy life. The lesson here is to show a willingness to take risks and go beyond your normal way of operating.

Yellow

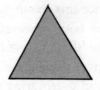

YELLOW–FIRST POSITION

This signifies the awakening of the conscious faculties in
Man, such as the five senses. You are likely to see life
through the focus of reason, logic and assessment,
depending on the mind constantly for information. You
are able to grasp things easily in an intellectual way,
calculating and analysing ceaselessly. You have a strong
tendency to be controlling and dominating and if you
don't get your own way, you can even be malicious and
vindictive. YELLOW people are usually good with words,
speaking fluently on matters which interest you. Speaking or lecturing on a given subject, or working with
words or numbers may be a perfect outlet. You generally
hold a position of responsibility and authority: you might
be a head of department, self-employed, a scientist or a
researcher. Generally, you enjoy the company of those
around you, especially when it is you who are the focus of
attention.

YELLOW – SECOND POSITION

This challenges you to consider not just your mental facility, but also your physical self. It is not uncommon for you to be lifted up into a world of fantasy, dreams, and imagination, neglecting the real, practical side of life. You need to get out of your conceptual mode. Your brilliant ideas may well be years ahead of their time, and the challenge will be to express your energy in a functional and creative way that has relevance in the present. This is often difficult for you, since you frequently lack patience, spreading your energies in many different directions at once, which leaves you frustrated and unfulfilled.

YELLOW – THIRD POSITION

You may need specific educational training to expand and open your mind. The subject to be studied must feel right to you and once the choice has been made, you should take positive, practical action to focus on the details – course of study, cost, duration, location – with thoroughness being of great importance. Taking this step, you will allow sunshine and light to prevail, bringing happiness and optimism into your life. What may be necessary at this time is a holiday, with lots of sun. The colour also indicates a need for you to use intellectual knowledge and understanding for service by teaching and educating people with whom you come into contact. Your service becomes more and more worthwhile as you tap into your innate intuition, allowing your potential power and natural wisdom to be channelled through you.

Green

GREEN–FIRST POSITION

You are neither dominating, nor submissive, extrovert nor introvert, but rather you seek balance and do not usually lean toward extremes of any kind. You often lack spontaneity, always deliberating before taking any action. You are usually very efficient and conscientious at work, and are neat and tidy in the home. GREEN people generally appreciate nature's beauty, are often drawn to parks, coasts, and open spaces. You usually surround yourself with plants and flowers both at home and work, whenever possible. You enjoy things that are made from wood, clay, and stone, and have an affinity to earthy, natural materials. You are able to vibrate a harmonious, soothing, gentle and sincere disposition. You do, however, tend to be overly cautious of life situations and people, and can find it difficult to break through the self-imposed barriers. It is important for GREEN people to regularly re-evaluate their attitude to life and consider the need for certain changes.

GREEN – SECOND POSITION

This challenges you to come to terms with emotional hurts. These can give rise to a deep sense of insecurity, leaving you ultimately disillusioned, bitter, envious, and jealous of other people. You may also feel a great sense of injustice, taking up causes in order to appease this feeling inside. On the surface your actions may appear worthwhile, but they usually stem from some unfulfilled need. You often feel threatened and vulnerable in life, constantly desiring protection. Often you find it difficult to share yourself, and tend to suppress your innermost feelings. You particularly hate the sensation of feeling enclosed, or trapped by confining and restricting situations. Your most important challenge is to encourage expression of your emotions at times when you feel most inclined to hold back.

GREEN – THIRD POSITION

You need to make contact with other people with whom you feel comfortable, developing new friendships and meaningful relationships. By expressing yourself like this you will see the value and benefit you can bring to others, and your basic sense of loss and alienation will be alleviated. You will no longer find life so serious and will start to experience more enjoyment: feelings of guilt, blame and general inertia which are typical qualities of GREEN, will begin to diminish. A general renewal of your outlook will start to blossom forth. This colour calls for alertness – being careful not to let situations pass by without making decisions.

Turquoise

TURQUOISE–FIRST POSITION

You have a basically sparkling youthfulness and bring imagination and fresh ideas to most situations. You usually project a calm and cool exterior, and are capable of dealing with demanding events. You have an attitude which allows you to 'take it in your stride' and you tend not to panic. TURQUOISE people are usually able to make decisions easily, and act with clarity. This usually makes you popular to be with, and to others you resonate with a sense of purpose and direction. You have a great deal of insight and talent and can use your abilities to further your own spiritual path. Essentially you are a good communicator and are able to express yourself easily. However, as the TURQUOISE personality is quite spiritually orientated, you frequently find it difficult to make your ideas a reality and overcome your tendency to be ungrounded.

TURQUOISE – SECOND POSITION

You must detach yourself from the crowd to maintain a healthy sense of identity, possibly because others feel drawn to your refreshing energy and will tend to make demands and invade your space. You must learn to create time away from other people in order to reflect inwardly. A process of cleansing and rejuvenating body, mind and emotions may be called for, due to over-indulgence and extremes of various kinds. This is your main challenge and since you are basically sensitive, toxification or illness may result if this challenge is ignored, causing disruption which can manifest itself in the body both internally and externally.

TURQUOISE – THIRD POSITION

You are able to see every life situation as a challenge. TURQUOISE encourages change and you are able to recognise that, although it often causes disruption and interference in your life, change is also the only constant quality. You usually welcome it, understanding that the action which must be taken is nothing less than a personal transformation (physical, emotional, mental and spiritual). This process frequently generates a vacuum of confusion, fear, turmoil and upset, and yet this is part of the process necessary for personal growth and development. Having moved through challenges and obstacles successfully, the rewards are always both uplifting and empowering. You are usually willing to 'have a go' – and the movement and the energy of TURQUOISE will help to elevate you to a new state of consciousness.

Blue

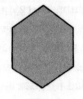

BLUE–FIRST POSITION

You are soft, gentle and peaceful by nature, rather than someone who is loud or easily excitable. You are generally considered to be passive and introverted, and usually spend much time dwelling on your inner spiritual self, seeking the meaning of your existence. Your essence works on a spiritual level, valuing qualities like truth and honesty. BLUE people tend to be trustworthy, reliable and faithful. People feel comfortable in your presence as you generate a non-threatening, serene, secure energy. However, you also have the tendency to be too self-absorbed. This often leads to isolation and inhibition, which ultimately causes you to lose confidence in yourself and your ability to cope with everyday situations. BLUE people seek order in their life and appreciate the constancy and reassurance of a framework or structure.

BLUE – SECOND POSITION

Your strength lies in your silence and your knowingness, not in your physical power as with RED people. Others see in you a stillness of mind and body. This peaceful appearance is the envy of all warm-spectrum people, but for you the challenge is to break through the silence which is so powerful within, and express more of yourself externally. Otherwise you will sink into the depths of melancholy and depression, and inertia, lethargy and further withdrawal will set in. The key is to come forward rather than withdrawing and hiding in isolation. You must develop your power of speech and self-expression, especially through the voice, in order to be able to develop as a whole human being.

BLUE – THIRD POSITION

Contemplation of spiritual and meditative matters, which come naturally to you, should be regarded as less crucial than a more earthly, realistic, practical attitude in the material plane. You must trust the process of life, and attend to seemingly ordinary, everyday matters. By doing so, you will find true beauty, freedom, and the spirituality you seek. Your key word is flexibility: you must be able to respond and participate in life without fear of being swallowed up by a 'big, bad world'. A period of rest, relaxation and tranquillity will be healing and satisfying to you, but it should be seen as a temporary measure, not as a means of permanent escape.

Violet

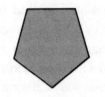

VIOLET–FIRST POSITION

Your basic essence is one of spiritual consciousness and awareness. You are usually interested in all aspects of the mystical and psychic forces which are beyond that of the physically explicable world. However you are usually more attuned to practical and earthly living than a BLUE person, since the colour VIOLET is itself created out of a marriage of RED and BLUE, and you therefore have the potential to apply your spirituality in a grounded way. You are willing to serve others in a worthwhile way, often in some form of healing. Within the VIOLET person, there resides a true dignity and nobility. You find it natural to express yourself aesthetically and artistically and you may be involved in the artistic professions, the Church, or in activities which have a degree of ceremony, high or fine quality extravagance or wealth. Healers and psychics are also to be found in this group. One of the weaknesses, however, of the VIOLET personality is that they often don't believe they can achieve their vision.

VIOLET – SECOND POSITION

You have the power to unite things and bring them together, and you are a natural leader, who is likely to be holding a position of authority. But, although you often accomplish things which others might find far too difficult, you usually also suffer from a fundamental emotional insecurity connected with your sense of self-worth and self-respect. The challenge for you is to ask for acknowledgement, recognition and honest feedback from those around you. The danger is that, if this feedback is not taken in, that you will retreat into a place of solitude, refusing to take responsibility in life (negative RED) and withdrawing into a process of escapism (negative BLUE). Others see this as immaturity or selfishness. So your challenge is to recognise that you have a particular purpose in life which must be fulfilled and not neglected under any circumstances. Maturity will only be gained through dedicated, active perseverance.

VIOLET – THIRD POSITION

Here, VIOLET encourages you to use your natural creativity and to share it with others. You have special healing qualities and need to practise using your innate capacity for faith, intuition and wisdom. 'Healing' does not mean that you have to be learned in any particular field of therapy, rather it may be pursued by applying these abilities in a general way. Be aware that you are not so spiritual that you are of no earthly use!

Magenta

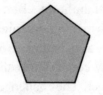

MAGENTA – FIRST POSITION

Your fundamental qualities are kindness, gentleness and consideration. You are usually affectionate and warm, showing compassion and love for others. You are often very mature, with a deep understanding of life, and you will instinctively encourage and guide others towards their full potential. MAGENTA people are co-operative, friendly, and genuine. You are often involved with work in the caring field, such as counselling, nursing or social work. Unconditional love and affection is a typical quality and you are sometimes described as 'the salt of the earth'.

MAGENTA – SECOND POSITION

There is a challenge for you to find a balance between giving and receiving in your life. You have a tendency towards giving others support and assistance, constantly encouraging them and pushing for the best for them. At the same time your own needs are often neglected, to your own detriment. The challenge is to learn that to receive is as valuable as to give, and that you don't have to give in return out of obligation or guilt. By meeting your own needs in this way, you can also show love and affection to yourself. This is as important to your life purpose as it is to help others. Nurture yourself and develop the ability to say 'no' when 'yes' would seem to be the easier way out.

MAGENTA – THIRD POSITION

You are able to blend the physical drive of RED and the spiritual lessons of VIOLET – a marriage between the first and seventh colours of the spectrum, and therefore a beautiful balance of the basic forces of life and of heavenly power. This blending has the potential to create an energy of enormous benefit to Mankind since it is the highest colour we can aspire towards in the physical world. It is a synthesis of the highest and the purest in human nature with the potential to create wholeness on a universal level. You are either striving towards this aim, or have reached it to some degree. The challenge is not to be caught up with the ego, or to develop a grandiose self-image, imagining yourself better than other people. In this case, an arrogant domineering and demanding nature will be revealed. You need to let go and allow the feminine and gentle part of yourself to come forth. Otherwise, you will feel a tendency to monopolise, manipulate and control, and this will keep you aloof, alone and distant from others.

Colour Reflection Readings

Reading 1

Beverley, a middle-aged woman, approximately 5ft 2in tall with medium build, had soft grey-blue eyes, a fair complexion and medium-brown hair. By profession she was a writer/journalist of Green issues and natural therapies. She was well-spoken, articulate and seemed very intelligent. Beverley had an engaging personality which was attractive and gave the feeling of being at ease. Her broad smile was very inviting, warm and friendly. When Beverley chose her colours she deliberated between each colour. She came wearing a BLUE-GREY sweat shirt, NAVY BLUE trousers and a NAVY jacket.

She took TURQUOISE as her first card, MAGENTA as her second, and BLUE as her third.

Interpretation

Turquoise This is the colour of clarity, bringing fresh, imaginative ideas into situations. Beverley had a constant need for clarity, and felt it important to stay young, open-minded and fresh in every area of her life. TURQUOISE is the colour created by the merging of BLUE and GREEN. For this reason, it is essentially cool and calming. Beverley had a sensitive and vulnerable nature. She tended to attract other people through what was seen as a sparkling personality, yet she needed time for her own reflection and solitude.

Magenta This is the eighth colour of our spectrum and is created from RED and VIOLET. It has a very deep spiritual quality and also shows that Beverley had a need for a nurturing and mothering energy and the tendency to be overly protective towards other people. We suggested that she find ways to meet these needs, and to experience receiving instead of always being the one to support and assist others in their lives. The main challenge for Beverley was to use her energy constructively, for herself.

Blue This colour implies an ultimate goal of inner and outward peace. It is a healing, spiritual energy to have around and would seem to reflect Beverley's inner desires. This colour hinted at her underlying need for withdrawal and rest. Beverley, at this point revealed that she was feeling inwardly depleted, and yearned for some time off to recuperate from the stresses of work. We pointed out that this rest was not to be seen as a form of 'retirement' or 'escapism', but as time for contemplation, to allow her to step out calmly and clearly in the material world. This was a time for consolidation, which would bring her closer to the TURQUOISE of her true nature.

Advice and action

The immediate need for Beverley was the colour MAGENTA, which took priority over the TURQUOISE and the BLUE since present circumstances indicated a negative level of MAGENTA at work. To realign and rebalance these energies and address the lack of fulfilment in Beverley's life at this time, it was essential that she incorporate MAGENTA more consciously. She was advised to wear regularly the MAGENTA spectrum in some way, perhaps by choosing a blouse, a scarf, a dress or nightgown, or bring the colour into her life through her bed-linen or her bath towels. She could try bringing flowers into her home. Pink roses and carnations of this colour are quite common and would help to remind her of her needs. Since MAGENTA is a nurturing colour, we advised Beverley to recognise and attend to her feminine needs by comforting and pampering herself and thereby show herself more love and compassion. She seemed to need permission in order to treat herself more lovingly. We recommended she take time off to have a full 'beauty treatment' so that she could incorporate and encourage the positive aspects of MAGENTA to work for her. We hoped that this would bring some colour into her life and put her 'in the Pink'.

After approximately three months we met Beverley again. 'It wasn't until I began receiving beauty-therapy treatment once a week,' she told us, 'that I realised how much replenishment I needed and how much I had let things go. Regularly attending the beauty clinic reminded me how much I needed MAGENTA.' By nurturing and nourishing herself in this way she brought the colour she needed most into her life which helped her to discover and appreciate her inner, feminine needs more.

'The PINK flowers in my home and the introduction of PINK items around me,' she went on, 'acted like a daily "memo", making me aware of my personal need for gentleness, softness, love and support. I feel so much more relaxed and more rested generally, and it shows in my work. When I sit down to write my mind is clear and free from the old cobwebs, and I can write more clearly and effectively.

'I am delighted with my Colour Reflection Reading and with the results of acting on your advice. I feel like a new person!'

Reading 2

Vanessa, a young mother, 24 years old, was separated and a single parent. She was petite and fragile with long, dark-brown hair, brown eyes and about 5ft 3in tall. She seemed weary and unsure of herself, but became excited and very attracted to the colours when they were laid out in front of her. On choosing her three colours she was very spontaneous and felt very satisfied with her choices. Vanessa wore a pale-BLUE cardigan, skin-tight, dark VIOLET leggings and a mixed-patterned autumnal-coloured skirt.

Vanessa's first choice was VIOLET, her second GREEN and her third ORANGE.

Interpretation

Violet Vanessa's first choice showed that her essence was basically spiritually inclined. She was potentially very powerful and able to remain balanced between her spiritual aspirations and her practical responsibilities. She often expressed her talents through art and creativity, but she needed to rely a great deal more on her intuition and to adopt a greater, more positive sense of self-worth, both of which are typically positive VIOLET qualities. At this time in her life, enhancing these qualities would be useful for Vanessa, as she was out of work and going through a divorce.

Green The GREEN colour reflected her need for space and personal freedom of expression, particularly the emotional hurt which seemed to exist as a result of past experiences. She confirmed that this was true and that it was reflected in her present state of being.

Vanessa wanted to know the best way for her to go forward, to allow her to contribute her natural talents and emphasise her own personal worth. Her baby might perhaps provide an opportunity to work in a positive and caring way. By focusing on her baby in this manner, we pointed out that she would be working on the positive level of GREEN, which would help her to develop aspects of herself which had slipped away, and which related to her sense of identity.

Orange   ORANGE as Vanessa's third choice revealed her courage and her constructive energy. As she moved towards this goal, this colour would give her the confidence to overcome obstacles in her life and add some vitality and much-needed zest to the quality of her life. It would also help Vanessa to move away from the trauma and depression she was currently experiencing.

Advice and action
What Vanessa needed to do was to get herself into some wide, open GREEN spaces – either in the countryside or even just a local park – allow herself to bask in the feeling of freedom, of being totally soothed and enveloped by the healing quality of nature. This would help her to see more clearly what should be the main priorities of her life and start to make decisions about them. By introducing this colour into her food and her clothes, and by surrounding herself with GREEN plants, she could begin to estab-lish an emotionally stable and balancing environment to support her. This colour would offer her emotional protection and help her to feel inwardly secure. We also advised Vanessa to bring the colour ORANGE (her third colour) into her life by means of ORANGE clothes, flowers like tiger lilies and chrysanthemums or ORANGE objects within her home. This would ensure that the negative aspects of GREEN – e.g. stagnation – would not prevail and, since she was already moving towards ORANGE, it was safe to recommend it.

After six months Vanessa came back to tell us how things had been developing for her. She told us of a trip she had taken to Ireland for ten days, spending time with her parents. There Vanessa became aware of the tremendous need she had for the colour GREEN and since Ireland is so well-known for its abundance of greenery she took full advantage of it! She went for long walks through the Irish countryside and could feel her worries drift away. It was on one of these walks that she decided she would look for a part-time job to earn some money, using her artistic and creative abilities and still have time to be with her daughter.

When Vanessa came to see us in November 1988 she hadn't found a suitable position, but she was confident that, because she now knew what she wanted, it would be much easier for her to find something. When we met five months later, Vanessa had found the 'perfect' job as a playgroup assistant, which meant that she didn't have to leave her daughter. It also provided a supportive environment to bring more ORANGE into her life by being around children.

Her divorce came through without complications, she had a new job, was earning a modest wage and had enough time to be with her daughter. As she put it, 'What more could I ask for? I've achieved so much in such little time already – who knows what's in store for me in the future?' She spoke with a real sense of hope and gratitude for the way things had worked out for her.

Reading 3

Robert, a prison officer, 28 years old and weighing approximately 13 stones, had a very strong and powerful physique. He seemed tense and stressed, but overall he was self-assured and confident. He had black hair and brown eyes with a pale complexion and was wearing a BLACK bomber jacket, BLACK trousers and a RED collared t-shirt when he came to see us.

Robert's first choice was RED, his second BLUE and his third YELLOW.

Interpretation

Red RED in the first position revealed that Robert was a basically outgoing and assertive individual. He had a strong, active attitude to life with an urgent desire for material success. He was warm and friendly, well liked by others, and could generally be relied upon to take responsibility in a practical way.

Blue This colour reflected his need for the release of stress and strain in his life. With an active nature, and a demanding and pressured job, Robert felt he had reached a saturation point within himself. He was desperately in need of replenishment, to recuperate his energies through some form of rest and relaxation. We suggested that he could gain temporary relief through meditation or prayer, and he was interested in finding out more about this.

Yellow   This colour indicated a desire for 'lightness' to help lift the depressive, heavy state of Robert's current situation. At the time he was unable to see the positive or optimistic side of life – and it was as if all colour had been drained from his expression of life. He needed to find a course or a direction which would help to raise his hopes and set him on a new and meaningful path. Since he was interested in finding out about various stress-releasing and self-help techniques, we recommended that he take such a course which would stimulate his mental attitude and give him a more positive outlook.

Advice and action

Robert's colour choice came predominantly from the warm end of the spectrum (RED in the first position and YELLOW in the third). It was therefore necessary for him to seek balance, especially with BLUE and to a lesser extent with TURQUOISE, from the cooler end of the spectrum. He was tired and stressed, and we advised him to adopt a less frantic pace in his life. Since BLUE was chosen as the second card, reflecting his present condition, we suggested surrounding himself with this colour. He could use it in his home, and, by wearing colours from the stronger tones in the spectrum, he could relax his over-active nature. Combined with the regular practice of stress-releasing skills, he would be able to create enough energy from the BLUE spectrum to balance himself successfully.

At the end of the reading, Robert said that initially he had been a bit sceptical, but he was amazed that three colours could reveal so much accurate information about his overall state. He left us with a greater sense of his whole situation and felt more hopeful.

Within a month of our having met Robert he decided to enrol on one of our courses. This and his CRR succeeded in motivating and stimulating his desire to overcome his general tiredness and lethargy. He now felt able to focus positively on his immediate situation.

The impact of the reading and the course encouraged Robert to refer several of his friends to us. They confirmed that he was much more pleasant and fun to be with – and had even enrolled on a meditation course!

chapter 2

■ ◆ ▲ ● ▼ ● ● ⬟

THE SUPER EIGHT COLOURS

To appreciate the nature of colour, let us look at the two very different ways in which colour theory has been historically approached – one by a great analytical scientist and the other by a poet and philosopher. Their contributions help us to establish both a scientific understanding of colour as well as a more intuitive and emotional response to it. They also help to establish a more balanced and workable system of colour theory for healing purposes, enabling us to appreciate why we use eight colours instead of seven.

The refraction of light was first described during the seventeenth century by Sir Isaac Newton. While experimenting with a prism, he noticed that it changed a beam of sunlight into narrow bands of colour creating a complete colour spectrum or, as it was later called, a 'rainbow'. He established that white light is a mixture of different light rays which are separated by the prism into seven major colours: RED, ORANGE, YELLOW, GREEN, BLUE, INDIGO and VIOLET (see Fig. 3 opposite). The seven colours seemed to fit perfectly alongside the seven basic notes in music and the seven major planets.

In 1706 he made the first known drawings of the colour circle, noting the similarity between VIOLET and RED, and linked them together forming the concept of a continuous circle of colour.

Johann Wolfgang Goethe, the philosopher, novelist and poet, published his own colour wheel in 1792, and in his monumental work of 1810 he elaborated his own theory of colour. Goethe's

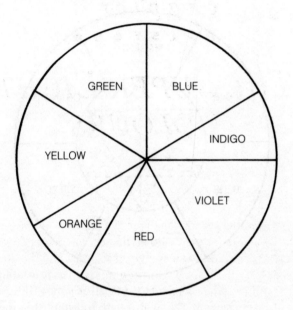

Fig. 3 Newton's Colour Wheel

colour wheel consisted of six colours: MAGENTA, ORANGE, YELLOW, GREEN, BLUE and VIOLET (see Fig. 4). Criticising Newton's approach to colour for its mathematical abstractions, he saw colour in terms of the dynamic flow of life, and stressed the importance of the experience of colour as a living sensation and an active interplay of light and darkness. For Goethe, colour was an expression of the essence of beauty, and Newton's observations seemed to him mechanical, static, and lacking in vitality.

Goethe's concern for the description of the energy of colour and its effects upon us, together with Newton's analytical observations, form the basis of contemporary colour theory. Neither Newton nor Goethe, however, offered us a colour wheel that is complete. Here are some of the differences between their two formulations:

- Newton saw RED as a pure form and included INDIGO in his spectrum;

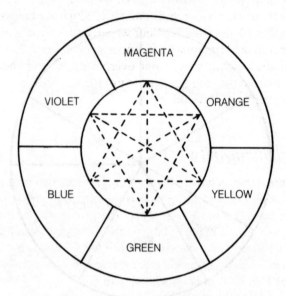

Fig. 4 Goethe's Colour Wheel

- Goethe omitted pure RED and INDIGO, and introduced MAGENTA (PEACH BLOSSOM);

- Newton's wheel was made up of seven different colours while Goethe's contains only six;

- Goethe's wheel introduced the concept of complementary colours; this would have been impractical for Newton, since his theory rested on an odd number.

Living Colour uses an eight-coloured spectrum enabling the idea of complementary colours to be an intrinsic part of the colour circle, as well as including a range of colours which contain equal amounts of warm and cool qualities. Using complementary colours brings a new dimension to our understanding of how colour works. It is in the light of this idea that both RED and its complementary colour, TURQUOISE, are included, in order to create a colour wheel that is harmonious and balanced.

This colour wheel is made of RED, ORANGE, YELLOW, GREEN, TURQUOISE, BLUE, VIOLET and MAGENTA, which are known as the Super Eight Colours. In this colour wheel, each colour is placed in a relationship of harmony with its opposite neighbour. It is important that the colours should not overpower or overwhelm one another: instead they are arranged to uplift each other, providing a balancing support all round.

Complementarity

Complementarity is based on one of the fundamental principles of the philosophy of Taoism, which is thousands of years old. The principle has been used to interpret the processes of nature and plays a vital role in Chinese medicine and astrology. Essentially the Chinese consider that life consists of two forces, opposing, but not antagonistic towards each other; these forces are known as Yin and Yang (see Fig. 5). Yin is associated with the feminine, Yang with masculine; Yin with expansion, Yang with contraction; Yin with night, Yang with day; Yin with cold, Yang with hot, and so on. Both forces move in cycles and are in constant change in relation to themselves and to each other due to the ebb and flow of the life forces of our universe.

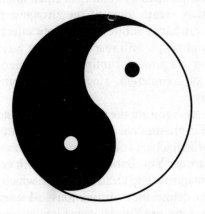

Fig. 5 Yin and Yang Symbol

To apply the principle of complementarity to colour we must
have an even number of colours to begin with, otherwise the
principle will not work. One colour would always be left without its
complement, as in the case of Newton's colour wheel. Although
Goethe used an even number of colours in his six colour wheel, he
omitted one of the most fundamental primaries, namely RED which
was an obvious introduction to our spectrum, since it is one of the
primary colours besides YELLOW, GREEN and BLUE. TURQUOISE
was also introduced because it is the perfect complement for RED.

TURQUOISE balances RED, neither submitting nor dominating in
relation to it. Through our work, we have come to see TURQUOISE
as a bridge between the physical and the spiritual planes, and at
this point in our evolution, TURQUOISE represents a reflection of a
new and growing movement towards self-development. It is
attuned with the changing ethos of the Age of Aquarius, which
brings with it the potential of mass awareness, especially regarding
personal and planetary growth.

INDIGO, a colour close to dark BLUE, is associated with self-
sacrifice: it reflects punishment and suffering, resulting in lack of
fulfilment, pain and martyrdom. The Piscean Age, which pre-
ceded the Age of Aquarius, has been a time of great trials, and of
great suffering. INDIGO, therefore, is a colour that has lost its
relevance to our spectrum, and in the mood of our society today as
a whole, we decided not to use it.

When two complementary colours of equal intensity are placed
side by side, they create some of the strongest possible colour
contrasts. This can have a subtle or a dramatic effect, depending on
the intensity, and people will react in varying ways ranging from
strong attraction to a powerful antipathy. Complementary colours
give an effect of completion, since they combine to present a
balanced energy.

Colours that are Yang are the warm colours of the spectrum and
those that are Yin are the cool ones. MAGENTA, RED, ORANGE, and
YELLOW are principally Yang colours and GREEN, TURQUOISE,
BLUE and VIOLET are Yin. Babbitt, the late 19th century chromo-
path, spoke of magnetic and electric colours, which may be seen as
another way to define their distinctions. Magnetic colours are
Yang, electric colours are Yin. However it must be said that within
both Yin and Yang, there exists its opposite. Therefore within Yin

there exists some element of Yang, and within Yang, there exists some Yin.

Each colour has its duality – its positive and negative qualities – which can either enhance or diminish or create lightness or darkness. For example, in the spectrum of REDS there are light ones and dark ones. Those REDS with more lightness can be considered as having more enhancing qualities, and are more Yin, while REDS with more darkness have more diminishing qualities and are therefore Yang in quality. Every colour has its complementary and therefore its cool and warm, passive and active counterpart.

When using colours therapeutically without the use of complementary colours, you can run risks of serious side effects. There are more chances of enhancing the problems you were aiming to relieve than actually relieving them. Let us suppose that you needed the colour RED because you were lacking in energy and vitality. You subject yourself to the colour RED in every way you can over a relatively long period of time, without using its complementary colour TURQUOISE to balance it. Sooner or later you will find yourself experiencing complete physical exhaustion and energy depletion due to being exposed to too much RED. In other words you 'overdosed' on the colour RED. Instead of RED giving you energy, it takes it away, drawing on your own energy resources. Using colours for therapeutic purposes without their complementaries to balance them tends to increase the chances of creating their opposite effects and clearly this would be counter-productive.

The Psychology of Colour

Scientific evidence suggests that light of different colours entering the eye can indirectly affect the centre of the emotions, via the hypothalamus and the pituitary, and despite the lack of conclusive scientific proof that colour influences the mind as it does the body, we cannot deny the fact that each of us in our own way responds to colour. For example, a BLUE that makes one person feel calm will be experienced as chilling to another; RED may be experienced as sensually evocative or extremely irritating.

In our experience, people tend to be attracted to certain colours according to a few overriding factors; their choice may be based on their personality type, the conditions of their life circumstances or their deep, possibly unconscious, innermost desires and thought processes. Some people will know exactly what colours they need, while others haven't a clue.

People do not necessarily choose a colour because it's good for them, but because they like the colour, even though it may be contrary to their needs. Why do people like specific colours? What is it that attracts or repels people to like or dislike specific colours? These colour responses may be traced back to childhood associations, or on reactions based on preference, or feelings against a symbolic or traditional meaning that have been attached to them. It may have to do simply with the changes of fashion or the flattering effects they create next to the skin.

Many psychological tests have been developed to help us discover about ourselves through the power of colour. Goethe believed that colour had an immediate effect on the emotions. Jung, who called the Yang principle the Animus and the Yin principle the Anima, believed in the symbolic power of colour and encouraged his patients to use colour spontaneously in paintings, to help them express the deepest unconscious part of their psyche and integrate it with the conscious to achieve wholeness.

Max Lüscher, who developed the 'Lüscher Colour Test' (see p. 10) while working on the effects of colours on the mind, believed that colours have emotional value and that a person's colour preferences reveal basic personality traits. A person's strong liking for RED indicates the assertive personality type, one who is outgoing and who has a strong will, while a dislike for this colour indicates a person who is shy and probably withdrawn from society.

In principle our colour-counselling work using the Colour Reflection Reading helps us to understand the physical, emotional and mental aspects of the individual. Information revealed and later discussed in depth often enables the person to integrate all these aspects of the complete personality. We are convinced that this technique is a powerful medium through which people can see themselves objectively and can wholistically improve their lives.

How the Super Eight Colours Affect Health

Each of the Super Eight Colours affects us on the emotional, mental and physical levels. You can add another dimension to your Colour Reflection Reading in Chapter 1 by relating it to the suggestions given in this section about the use of colour energy in correcting imbalances. These are simple ways of using colour for healing.

Take your colour choices from the Colour Reflection Reading and check the section on those colours. Be intuitive and spontaneous when recognising strengths and weaknesses, and exploring the enhancing or diminishing aspects. Use these concepts to acknowledge strengths and isolate and define weaknesses in your state of health. You will then be able to make basic changes, using the other chapters in this book, bringing colour into your life in a positive and practical way. Bear in mind that a diminishing aspect is often the opposite of an enhancing one. Thus an enhancing quality of RED is willingness to act. The opposite (unwillingness to act) is a diminishing aspect.

Mental and Emotional Qualities of Red
(complementary colour – TURQUOISE)

Enhancing aspects
RED, the first colour of the spectrum, speaks of motivation, stimulation, activity and will. It brings new life and new beginnings. Its energy is primal, compared with the other colours. It is associated with warmth and excitement, with initiative and willingness to act, and with the pioneering spirit that lifts us up. Persistence, physical strength, drive and power are typical traits. Friendliness and forgiveness are two beautiful qualities of this colour, as are prosperity and gratitude. Physical love and carnal passion are synonymous with RED.

Diminishing aspects
Indecency and coarseness, a lack of refinement, and a certain obstinacy may begin to operate here. Physical cruelty, grossness and danger may become evident. RED's intrinsic intensity and

force can develop into anger and fiery rage, or may be expressed as brutality, ruthlessness, resentment or revolt.

Physical Effects of Red

RED is a warm colour with an extrovert character. It stimulates vitality and energy throughout a living organism, and where there is sluggishness, it promotes activity. RED gets the adrenalin going, assists the blood's circulation within the body, and helps in the manufacture of haemoglobin for new RED blood cells. RED raises blood pressure, promotes heat in the body, and stimulates the nervous system, which is why it can be used so effectively to treat various forms of numbness and paralysis. Anaemia, colds, and pneumonia are other disorders which can be alleviated by RED.

RED lends vigour to the physical functions, and relieves inertia, melancholy, sadness, depression and lethargy. RED carries the energy which is needed for building and strengthening the body. It is especially useful for those 'run-down' times or for low resistance. RED acts as a tonic and can overcome the first signs of a chill. In cases of chill, a practical way to introduce RED energy is by wearing RED socks or gloves and a RED vest or a scarf. Another excellent way to warm the body and stimulate energy internally is with regular practice using the colour breathing, colour visualisation and meditation exercises for the colour RED (see Chapter 7).

RED is not recommended in the treatment of fever, hypertension, or any inflammatory conditions such as swellings, open wounds, burns or bruises.

Mental and Emotional Qualities of Orange
(complementary colour – BLUE)

Enhancing aspects
ORANGE is outgoing and assertive, as is RED, but it is more constructive. ORANGE reflects enthusiasm, with a natural, impulsive vivaciousness. This colour brings the 'kiss of life': good health, vitality, creativity and joy, as well as confidence, courage, buoyancy, spontaneity and a positive attitude to life. Communication, movement and enterprise are often features of this colour, and its finest attribute is bliss.

Diminishing aspects

The adverse side of ORANGE can involve an overbearing or overwhelming attitude. This may be expressed in flamboyance or an exhibitionistic streak. The negative vibrations of ORANGE are associated with joylessness, melancholy and sadness, and at its extreme may be reflected in loss of vitality, despondency and destructiveness.

Physical Effects of Orange

The energy of this colour has some basic similarities with RED and YELLOW, stimulating the blood and circulatory processes, and affecting the mental and nervous and respiratory systems. ORANGE energises the body, and assists in the assimilative and distributory processes. It is the colour of calcium, and is recommended for pregnant women and mothers who wish to encourage the generation of breast milk for feeding. Healthy hair, nails, bones and teeth are produced with this colour. ORANGE can be used for the treatment of the spleen and for kidney disorders.

For example, this colour could be introduced into your system by wearing it anywhere from your middle to the lower part of the body, either in a shirt or trousers, or even underwear. It affects the physiological functioning of the stomach, pancreas, bladder and lungs, and relieves ulcers and gallstones. It is especially effective in relieving wind and gases from the body, and brings balance to those who suffer intestinal cramps and a sluggish or spastic colon. Constipation can also be treated effectively with the colour ORANGE.

ORANGE promotes a stronger heartbeat, and is helpful to the liver. It is therefore a good colour for the treatment of alcoholics. With its effect on the respiratory system, it is also valuable in treating bronchitis, encouraging deep, rhythmic breathing. Some of the lighter tints of this colour may be used in treating arthritis and rheumatism.

ORANGE is not a colour for people who are easily irritated or suffering from stress.

Mental and Emotional Qualities of Yellow
(complementary colour – VIOLET)

Enhancing aspects

YELLOW is the 'lightest' of all the warm-spectrum colours and the colour which most resembles the sun. It brings with it hope, and the feeling that everything will be all right. It has an air of radiance, brightness, cheerfulness and gaiety. YELLOW is open-minded and inspiring; it glows and illuminates, and at its most positive vibration it corresponds with knowledge and wisdom. Reason and logic flow from it, and intellectual discrimination, discernment, and decisiveness all resonate with it.

Diminishing aspects

The negative vibration of YELLOW can be extremely destructive. It involves deception, deviousness, controlling behaviour, calculation, maliciousness, vindictiveness and flattery. It can lead to an extreme negativity associated with mental depression and deep pessimism.

Physical Effects of Yellow

YELLOW works to strengthen the nervous system and the muscles, including the heart, creating better circulation. It assists in stimulating various bodily functions, such as the action of the liver, the gallbladder, and the flow of bile. YELLOW promotes secretion of gastric juices, and relieves constipation and indigestion by promoting proper bowel movement. It is an excellent colour for the relief of inflammatory disorders of the joints and connective tissues and can alleviate arthritis, rheumatism and gout.

A practical way to apply YELLOW energy is with regular practice using the colour breathing, colour visualisation and meditation techniques in Chapter 7. Focus on the affected areas by directing colour energy towards them. Or sit in the sun's rays for a while on a regular basis if possible and soak up the radiant GOLDEN YELLOW rays whenever you can.

YELLOW has the capability of loosening calcium deposits within the system, and so it is effective in relieving stiffness of the joints, and pain experienced during movement. It is also a purgative, and works exceptionally well to stimulate the kidney and the liver, and dispels mucus from the body. It can cleanse the bloodstream and activate the lymphatic system. YELLOW helps diabetics lower their daily intake of insulin, and encourages the natural flow of pancreatic insulin. Iodine, phosphorus, gold and sulphur all contain this YELLOW energy.

Although YELLOW is a colour which stimulates the brain and the mental faculties, it is not recommended for anyone suffering from severe mental illness or neurosis.

Mental and Emotional Qualities of Green
(complementary colour – MAGENTA)

Enhancing aspects
The energy of GREEN reflects sharing, adaptability, generosity and co-operation. It soothes the emotions, invites good judgement, conscientiousness and understanding. It is the image of security and protection and creates an environment appropriate for making decisions. Space, freedom, harmony and equilibrium all stem from GREEN's natural sense of justice. GREEN acts as a signal for the renewal of life, and its highest vibration reflects the spirit of evolution.

Diminishing aspects
Miserliness, indifference and insecurity are some of GREEN's negative expressions. Poor judgement, over-cautiousness and suspicion are represented in GREEN's negative nature, and, together with precociousness, it can indicate jealousy, envy, selfishness and prejudice. At its lower levels GREEN fosters stagnation and ultimately degeneration.

Physical Effects of Green

GREEN is particularly beneficial for the sympathetic nervous system and it is useful for general healing, balancing and cell restoration. GREEN is related to the heart and has a direct effect on the function of the heart and the lungs. It dissolves blood clots and relieves stagnation and hardening of the cells. GREEN assists the building of .

muscles, skin and tissues. It also aids the elimination of toxic material and acts as a mild astringent.

GREEN will relieve tension, and can lower blood pressure. It has a relaxing, sedative effect, although if used wrongly it can bring on drowsiness, tiredness or irritability.

Since this colour is capable of influencing the basic cell structure, it can be used to treat tumours, cysts and growths. It is especially good for chest complaints such as asthma, chronic bronchitis and angina. If you are feeling physical constriction in your chest area, try the breathing exercise explained in the colour breathing and colour visualisation section and the GREEN meditation in Chapter 7. This will help you open and expand your chest and let go of tightness. Regular visits to your local parks, or to the countryside for a 'breath of fresh air' will also do you good.

GREEN is also used for inflammatory liver conditions, colds and headaches. Since GREEN acts as a balancing force, it alleviates fear in traumatic situations, and is effective in treating shock. It also helps people who suffer from claustrophobia.

Mental and Emotional Qualities of Turquoise
(complementary colour – RED)

Enhancing aspects
TURQUOISE has a constant vibrancy which neither overpowers nor intrudes in any way. It has an aura of alertness and awareness which gives great clarity of expression. This sparkling, articulate colour has an attentive, open-minded quality which emanates well-being. It is liberal, helpful and triumphant. Fresh TURQUOISE offers the opportunity for change and ultimately, transformation at its highest level.

Diminishing aspects
TURQUOISE can sometimes be plagued by an immaturity which can manifest confusion and an inability to get further on in life. Isolation and separation are further negative attributes, with feelings of emptiness and lack of clarity on an emotional, spiritual and mental level.

Physical Effects of Turquoise

TURQUOISE is created by combining BLUE and GREEN. It is a wonderfully cool, relaxing and refreshing colour which aids any inflammatory condition such as headache, swellings, cuts, bruises or burns. Next time you burn or cut yourself, immediately place your hand on the affected area (or have another person do it for you) while you send the anti-inflammatory colour TURQUOISE directly towards it (see p. 141). Using the colour breathing and the colour visualisation techniques and the TURQUOISE meditation from Chapter 7, you can create an image of the wound becoming calmer and less active.

TURQUOISE is especially good for skin problems, including acne, eczema and psoriasis. It relieves stress and tensions, and helps to remove toxic waste and congestion from the body.

TURQUOISE works on the immune system, acting as a protection against invasion by harmful bacteria and viruses. Colitis, dysentry and fevers are especially responsive to TURQUOISE, which also assists the elimination process. It helps to clear sinuses, mental fatigue and hay-fever. It replenishes the whole system. In fact the colour TURQUOISE is the colour which seems to be the most popular with AIDS sufferers, especially in the early stages of the dis-ease.

TURQUOISE is not recommended for people with sluggish or underactive conditions.

Mental and Emotional Qualities of Blue
(complementary colour – ORANGE)

Enhancing aspects
BLUE marks the entry into the deeper realms of the spirit, and one of its finest qualities is aspiration. BLUE is part of the cool spectrum, and in its stillness and faith this colour promotes devotion and trust. It is a popular colour, associated with duty, beauty and tact. BLUE's serenity brings with it peace, faith and lovely relaxing, healing feelings. Its fluidity and quiet strength are attractive traits, which evoke admiration from others.

Diminishing aspects
The BLUE nature searches and seeks continually. Common aspects of the negative vibration of BLUE are doubt and disbelief, and lack

of tact. It is unrealistic and promotes daydreaming, tending towards sloppiness, complacency and distrust. From tiredness, laziness and dullness, BLUE can move into a melancholic state, finally attracting a total sense of inertia.

Physical Effects of Blue

BLUE has a calming, relaxing effect. It is the antidote to RED and is used successfully to treat feverish conditions, fast pulse rate, and high blood pressure. Generally, it will reduce heat and inflammation from the body, such as sunburn or sunstroke cases. It will promote serenity and release from tension, stress and headache, and relieves all throat or vocal imbalances, such as sore throats, coughs, hoarseness and laryngitis (see also p. 145).

It has been used effectively to treat menstrual imbalances such as period pains, backache, or even blood flow. Women with menstrual problems can use the healing quality of the colour BLUE immediately before, during and after periods. BLUE nightwear, panties and bathrobes as well as BLUE clothes for the daytime can be considered, and household items like bed-linen and towels can all help relieve menstrual imbalances. A BLUE light left on over night can also help to relieve and reduce menstrual tension and pain.

Other imbalances for which BLUE would be useful are migraine, meningitis, colitis, dysentry, insomnia and diarrhoea. BLUE is especially good for children's ailments, such as teething, throat troubles, tonsilitis, measles, whooping cough, chicken pox and hiccups. Many eye troubles can be resolved with BLUE, including myopia (short-sightedness), cataracts, and photophobia (sensitivity to light).

BLUE is not advised when treating paralysis, low blood pressure, or colds. Neither is it recommended for melancholia or depression.

Mental and Emotional Qualities of Violet
(complementary colour – YELLOW)

Enhancing aspects
This colour, combining both BLUE and RED, reflects dignity,

nobility and self-respect. It is the colour of royalty and, at its most sublime, vibrates with the power of integration and oneness. When its innate quality is aligned through psychic energy with vision and intuition, it is the author of destiny. Artistry, tolerance and consideration are associated with VIOLET. Its soothing, calming power represents a practical idealism informed with humility.

Diminishing aspects

The negative side of VIOLET includes forgetfulness and lack of endurance. Inconsiderateness, disrespect and an argumentative, demanding attitude spring from misuse of this energy. It can degenerate into impractical idealism, separateness, corruption and disintegration. Pride and arrogance are also present at this level.

Physical Effects of Violet

VIOLET normalises all glandular or hormonal activity, as it is connected to the function of the pituitary gland at the base of the brain. It works well for cerebro-spinal meningitis, concussions, epilepsy and any other mental or nervous disorders such as obsessional disorder and personality imbalances. VIOLET will relieve neuralgia and problems associated with the eyes, ears and nose. Regular practice of colour breathing and colour visualisation exercises using VIOLET can encourage greater movement and flexibility of the eyes and strengthen weak eyes.

VIOLET is especially valuable as a blood purifier and assists the building of leucocytes (WHITE blood cells). VIOLET helps to keep a balance of sodium and potassium in the body, which in turn helps to regulate water balance and normalise heart rhythms. The lungs, liver and kidneys may also be treated successfully with this colour. Sciatica and general nervous disorders are helped by VIOLET.

Mental and Emotional Qualities of Magenta
(complementary colour – GREEN)

Enhancing aspects

Most refined and subtle of all the colours, MAGENTA transmutes desire into its physical equivalents. Dedication, reverence, gratitude and commitment are ascribed to this colour, as it strives to express idealism in its purest form. MAGENTA is the last of the colours, bringing with it a high degree of understanding and maturity as a consequence of its passage through all the other colours. Administrative ability is characteristic here, together with great compassion. MAGENTA is a gentle, warm, nurturing and protective colour, and unconditional or spiritual love is its highest expression.

Diminishing aspects

This side of MAGENTA can create the energy of superiority, which tends to lead towards snobbishness, arrogance, and ultimately, isolation. Adverse aspects of MAGENTA can result in a dominating, monopolising and fanatical outlook. Lack of self-love, non-appreciation of personal needs, and insecurity are all within the range of MAGENTA here. Self-esteem that is out of proportion can result in misuse of this colour's inherent knowledge and power.

Physical Effects of Magenta

This colour increases the blood supply to the brain and stimulates the sympathetic nervous system. It relieves headaches, head colds, high blood pressure and chronic tiredness or nervous breakdown.

If you have a tendency towards over-exertion, try wearing the colours MAGENTA or PINK. One appropriate way to receive the energy of MAGENTA would be to treat yourself to some kind of relaxation, such as a massage or a holiday period. MAGENTA is also especially good for amnesia and for comas. MAGENTA helps the function of the heart, including disorders such as heart murmurs, palpitations, and 'heartburn'. The energy of this colour is gentle, soothing and protective. It aids expansive breathing, energises the adrenal glands and the kidney areas, and can also be used as a diuretic. MAGENTA can act as a stabiliser for the emotionally disturbed, and in cases where there may be aggressive or violent behaviour.

chapter 3
■ ◆ ▲ ● ▼ ⬟ ● ●

YOUR AURA COLOURS

This chapter is about the subtle bodies around the physical body, i.e. the electromagnetic field known as the aura. The electromagnetic spectrum includes both the visible colours and a wide range of non-visible energy. The whole spectrum is largely a product of the sun's rays, which envelop the earth and endow all living things with radiant energy. It is this field which gives rise to the aura.

We will also look at the chakra system which relates to the Super Eight Colours and which represents those major points or power centres of the human body through which colour energy is able to enter and leave and together reflect the overall state and condition of a person's state of health – physically, emotionally and mentally.

To illustrate how the aura and the chakra systems work together and influence us, here is a common situation which most of you have probably experienced yourselves. Consider the situation when you have heard some bad news which causes you distress, or you've found yourself in a situation which causes you to feel anxiety (such as taking exams, going for a job interview, appearing on stage or giving a talk, etc). To one degree or another you have probably felt a churning, spinning or flapping (butterfly) sensation in the region of your lower abdomen. This type of experience is the expression of the chakra located at the navel region which predominantly absorbs the colour YELLOW and can be seen in the aura as vibrating more powerfully than the other spectrum colours. YELLOW is also the colour which is associated with the nervous system and is linked with our thought processes. So when we are concerned, feeling anxious or upset as described above, this chakra begins to respond actively, indicating a movement of energy in this part of the body. This movement of energy is the expression of dissipation or disorientation of energy. Clairvoyants can see these movements of energy in the aura while others can feel them.

We recall our own situation when we were to give a talk in front of approximately 200 people, which was also to be recorded for television. Although we had over the years given many talks and lectures this was the first time we were to be filmed. It was clearly an important occasion for us and we felt extremely excited but also nervous about it. Both our chakras at the navel region flapped every time we thought about it days before, and on the day itself, when the time came to give the talk we could feel each other's nervousness from a distance. Being so aware of what was happening we were consciously able to calm and de-energise the negative effects and thus not be overpowered and controlled by what was going on in our bodies on a deeper level. The most effective means we could use at the time was to breathe deeply and visualise a relaxing and restful soft BLUE-WHITE light, bathing us from top to bottom, as if a shower of light were pouring down on us from above. On the out-breath it was important to release as fully as possible any tension that we were feeling. This we found worked extremely well and helped us before, during and after the talk, which turned out to be a great success.

The Electromagnetic Spectrum

The part of the electromagnetic spectrum with which we are concerned in this book is the visible portion, i.e. white light and colour.

It was Newton who established that white light is a mixture of different light rays, which are separated by the prism into seven major colours – RED, ORANGE, YELLOW, GREEN, BLUE, INDIGO, VIOLET. These rays – or wavelengths – move at different speeds.

At one end of the visible spectrum, where the wavelengths are extended and slow, we see the colour RED. At the other end, where the wavelengths are shorter and faster moving, we can observe the more refined, less dense colours such as BLUE and VIOLET. Wavelengths found on either side of this visible part of the spectrum include infrared and ultraviolet as well as radio waves, gamma rays, X-rays and cosmic rays. (See Fig. 6.)

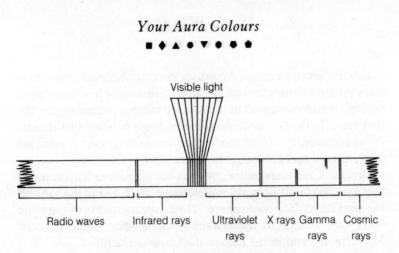

Fig. 6 *The Electromagnetic Spectrum*

The Aura

All matter is constantly exchanging vibrations of different wavelengths. These vibrations affect us even though they may not be visible to the eye, and we may not be conscious of their existence. The part of the electromagnetic spectrum which surrounds us and penetrates us represents our 'aura'.

Colour energy doesn't just express the way we think, feel and act, it also reflects back to us from the external environment, either raising or lowering our spirits. All changes, whether mental, emotional, physical or spiritual in nature, are connected with changes which take place in the electromagnetic field that is in us and around us. Each of us creates his or her own magnetic atmosphere, and this unfailingly reveals the nature of our disposition, temperament, character and our state of well-being. Thus a person lacking the colour RED in their aura may express this mentally and emotionally with a lack of drive or initiative in their life, and physically by suffering from low blood pressure. On the other hand a person with an excess of the colour RED would probably tend to express themselves more overtly than inwardly.

In our language we constantly use phrases like 'RED with rage', 'GREEN with envy', 'feeling BLUE', 'BROWN study', 'in the PINK', etc., in order to express how we feel or how we see others. Perhaps without consciously realising, we are actually responding to the colour/s of our own or other people's auras.

Edgar Cayce, a famous American psychic, believed that a person's preference for a certain colour revealed his or her major 'aura colour', which explained the reason for being attracted to it in the first place. In the Colour Reflection Reading a person's first choice, i.e. their favourite colour tends to represent their overall spiritual development and predominant aura colour at that time.

Greeks, Christians and Egyptians have believed for centuries that man sends out light at a microcosmic level, just as the sun and the stars do in their own sphere. Their representation of the auric body can be seen in the elaborate and elegant headdresses of Egyptian art, and in the halo of the Christian saints.

Many people have the ability to see the aura around a person, even though it may only be glimpsed momentarily. Perhaps without realising it we 'feel' auras more frequently than we actually see them. How many times for instance, have you seen a stranger walk into a room and have the sense that although you've never met before, you have an immediate feeling for that person? You find yourself gravitating towards that person like iron filings to a magnet. On the other hand a different person enters the room and you share very little interest, if any. You may even feel repelled and feel the need to withdraw.

The aura is like an antenna, capable of receiving information and sending out messages. Each of us can learn to become more sensitive to 'pick up' vibrations from auras. In fact this can be heightened and developed with practice. As we develop, we become more aware of the interchange of energies surrounding ourselves and other people. By practising various meditational exercises and learning to trust your intuitional response to everyday situations and circumstances, you can develop your ability to interpret what you see and feel, and monitor each others' auras.

Proof the Aura Exists

Many clairvoyants and psychics are sensitive to the energies emanating from the physical body, and are able to use this sensitivity as a tool for healing and diagnosis. But while occultists, clairvoyants and psychics have always been quite clear about the existence of the aura, many physicians and scientists traditionally have looked on the idea with scepticism.

Dr Walter J. Kilner, of St Thomas's Hospital, London, developed a screen which was sensitive to the normally invisible energy of the ultraviolet spectrum, and was able to show the existence of vaporous energy in the form of bands of light extending away from the body. Auras could be seen and believed by anyone who doubted the reality of these human emanations.

Semyon and Valentina Kirlian, two Russian experimenters, succeeded in taking photographs of the energy fields around various objects. Although Kirlian photography does not record the aura in its entirety, it provides us with a 'picture' of the emanations nearest to the physical body. These photographs use an electric current to reveal and record the patterns of energy that shoot out from the body. The texture and the composition of this energy varies from person to person. Rays of light shoot out at right angles and at regular intervals all around the body, sometimes gently, at other times pulsating quickly. These rays also extend out to different lengths both horizontally and vertically. The longest rays normally emanate from the fingers, knees, elbows and hips.

The aura, skin response and brain response seem to be involved with colour through electrical impulses, which the human body generates in most parts. The series of electrical and magnetic emissions expressed by the physical body can be measured with modern equipment such as the electroencephalograph (EEG), which measures brainwaves. (This literal translation from the Greek is 'a picture of electrical impulses inside the brain'.) Today with such advances in scientific approaches, we are able to confirm the wisdom of psychics and mystics with modern scientific technology.

Exercises to Help You Feel Your Subtle Energies

1. Sit or stand comfortably.

2. Place your hands approximately 12 ins apart and hold this position for a minute or so and breathe normally.

3. Slowly begin to move your hands closer together to approximately 6–8 ins apart and then pause.

4. Now slowly move your hands further apart to about 10–12 ins and then pause. Slowly move your hands back and forth,

increasing and decreasing the space between your hands and notice what you feel. As you increase the distance between your hands it should feel something like stretching a piece of elastic; as you decrease the space, the pressure is built up or the elastic stretch is reduced.

5. Now move your hands together until the fingers are almost touching each other. Leave about 1¼in between them and notice your experience.

Many people experience prickling sensations, some fine and gentle, others strong and coarse. Some people report experience of intense heat, while others feel cool or cold tickling sensations. Whatever your experience with this exercise, even if what you felt between your hands was minimal, it just goes to show we do not stop at our skin.

Here is an exercise you can practise with one other person.

1. Stretch your hands out towards each other leaving a distance of about 8 in between you and hold for a moment.

2. Decide who will go first and then gently push and pull, let's say the left hand to start with, until the other can feel the energy received in the palms or fingers of their right hand. Ensure that the hands do not touch. Notice what it feels like to move this energy and to receive it.

3. Now the other person should try to do the same. When both of you have done this with your left hand, try it with your right. See if you feel through which hand your partner is directing vital energy to you.

It might be worth mentioning that some people feel the energy in their fingers, while others feel it in the palms of their hands. There is no incorrect way to feel this energy. What is important is that you feel it. Do not worry, however, if at first you do not feel anything. Keep trying. The more you practise the more sensitive you will become and gradually the more you will feel, even if it's only a little bit.

The Function and Composition of the Aura

The word aura comes from the Greek word *avra* meaning 'breeze'. The complete aura is experienced as an ovoid orb of subtle emanations surrounding the physical body.

One of the main functions of the aura is to absorb 'white' light from the atmosphere, divide it into its component colour energies – RED, ORANGE, YELLOW, GREEN, TURQUOISE, BLUE, VIOLET and MAGENTA – and direct these to the appropriate power centres or chakras within the physical body. This process helps to maintain our good health, restore balance where disease may be starting, and also encourage the release of toxic materials or waste products which the body no longer needs. The action of the chakras is described more fully on p. 72.

The aura is directly related to the chakras, and the colours expressed in the aura and the chakras directly relate to each other. Where a person's aura colours radiate and glow vibrantly, the correlating chakras absorbing those colours will radiate and glow as well. The opposite is also true.

In an evolved individual, the predominant colour of the aura will be VIOLET or MAGENTA. This means that the Third Eye or Crown chakras, which directly relate to VIOLET and MAGENTA, are the strongest and most active. A less developed individual will carry the primal colour of RED. Generally, the more developed the individual, the more extended their aura will be. It is said that the extent of the aura, and its general condition, is related to the development of the mind and soul of the individual in question. In a healthy person, the colours of the aura are vital and clean, without 'perforations' (see Fig. 7 on p. 66).

Tiredness and physical depletion will affect the vitality of the aura. When a person's aura is 'out-of-balance' or will not emanate clear or true colours, it may give out dull, pale or greyish colours instead. Dark shades, with flecks, patches or 'arrow' shapes can appear in the affected areas. Breaks in the aura will also appear indicating energy 'leaking' from the body at those points. Individuals who smoke or drink heavily usually show depleted auras, with all these signs (see Fig. 8 on p. 67).

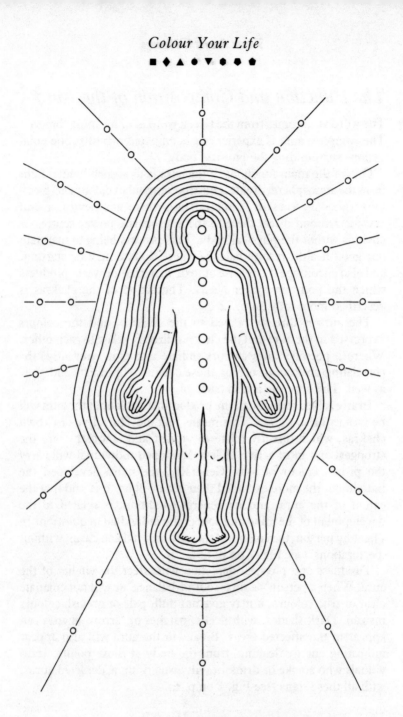

Fig. 7 A Healthy Aura

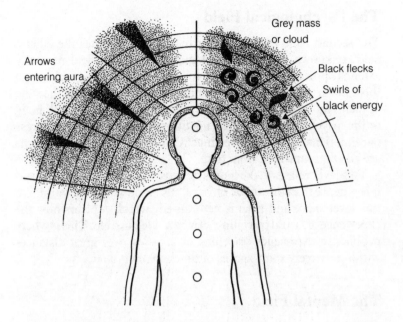

Fig. 8 An Afflicted Aura

The aura is made up of three major layers extending outwards from the body, and these have three major functions: to protect, to absorb, and to communicate.

The Etheric Field

The first band of energy, which penetrates the physical body, is known as the 'etheric' field and is sometimes referred to as the 'matching' body. It is the medium through which life-sustaining energy flows from the sun and the planets, from the atmosphere around us, and from the distant cosmos. This field is normally about 3–4 ins wide and acts as a protective layer around our physical selves. Often it is seen as a glow of light BLUE or SILVERY light emanating around the physical body, especially around the head and shoulders. Along with the physical body it represents the three-dimensional world on the material plane. It is the lowest of the auric fields and has the most dense vibrations, more solid and manifested than any of the other succeeding layers.

The Psychological Field

The second band of radiation, which interpenetrates the etheric field, is known as the 'psychological' aura. This field normally extends approximately 2–4 ft beyond the physical body, although this can vary according to each individual, depending on the state of their emotions. This body is also referred to as the 'astral' body or the 'psychic' body. It is the medium through which we express our emotions and sensate feelings. Our fears, hopes and passions are all communicated from here.

This layer relates to the fourth dimension and its vibrational field is less dense than that of the physical, three-dimensional world. On this level space and time is neutralised, which explains how the experience of 'astral travelling' can be made possible. This is where people can experience travelling or crossing over great distances within relatively short spaces of time – *in an instant*.

The Mental Field

The third band of the aura is called the 'mental' body or the 'spiritual' aura, and interpenetrates the 'psychological' field. This body is chiefly concerned with our thought processes and the type of thoughts we construct and express, both in concrete and in abstract form. This body extends to a distance of about 8 ft and sometimes even further, depending on the individual. It is in constant movement and its colour and texture are finer and more subtle than either the 'psychological' aura or the 'etheric' field.

This layer is related to the fifth-dimensional world and unlike the other two layers, space and time is transcended within this dimension. It is through this layer that we can begin to connect spiritually with other beings or souls, and with the greater universe.

Double-Etheric Fields

Between each of the three basic layers of the aura, there are further vibrational levels. These levels are known as the 'double-etheric' fields, which exist as corresponding fields to link each level with the next. They supply life-giving energy to each of the layers and sustain them. These levels might be compared with FM radio waves, since they are ceaselessly modulating in frequency as they send out and receive information. The double-etheric fields are just like the membranes of our cell walls, in that these are 'semi-porous', working in both directions to let oxygen and nutrients in, and allow carbon dioxide and waste products out.

The three bodies which comprise the aura are like the subtle garments worn by the Spiritual Being to express itself. Together they make up the complete personality and can exist independently from one another.

When a person dies and departs from the physical, material world, the double-etheric disintegrates and the process of trans-formation from the physical world to the psychic world takes place. In fact the double-etheric begins the process of disintegration and degeneration well before death is imminent. During the period leading up to serious ill-health on the physical level, the etheric bodies struggle to survive and maintain themselves to keep the physical body functioning as normally as possible. If the illness is not alleviated, the over-burdened etheric fields eventually weaken and lose all strength to protect the physical body, which will eventually cease to function.

The Ozone Layer and the Etheric Field

The Ozone Layer which surrounds the Earth and protects all living organisms within it could be described as the etheric field of the Earth's crust, similar to the etheric field of the human body. Ozone is a gas closely related to oxygen, which helps to keep the Earth's atmosphere balanced and thereby serves as a vital function to life. If this important layer is depleted or punctured in any way, similar to the etheric field of the human body, it becomes vunerable and it lets in the harmful ultraviolet rays. (In such instances scientists have been warning us of the 'Greenhouse Effect'.)

Seeing Auras

One autumn evening in 1981 Howard and I went for a walk and decided to stop at a pub for a glass of sherry to warm ourselves up before making our way home. As we were sitting there, I saw in the distance, above the head and shoulders of a fairly young woman with black hair, some jagged BLACK and murky GREY arrows and specks which appeared to hover in mid air between about 6–12 ins from her body.

At first I thought it must be the sherry! But since my glass was not even half-way empty, I decided it must be something else. I looked again and tried to focus on what was happening, and then it dawned on me that what I was seeing was an afflicted aura. At the time my knowledge about auras was very limited and I had never experienced seeing one. I had felt it many times, but not seen it.

Initially it seemed that the harder I tried to see it, the more difficult it became. The specks in the woman's aura seemed to fade and then suddenly to reappear. What seemed like ages turned out to be only a few seconds. As I focused more on what I saw, I experienced the BLACK and GREY specks and arrows moving aggressively, pulsating both inwardly and outwardly, to and from her physical body. They were surrounded with a mass of dull GREY cloud which gave me the feeling of a lot of heaviness and congestion.

Howard by this time was wondering why I wasn't paying him any attention. I pointed out the lady and he discreetly turned round to see for himself, but was unable to see what I saw. We both noted that the woman was a smoker and the table where she sat was filled with empty half-pint beer glasses obviously drunk by the man she was with, and her own empty wine glasses. On closer observation the woman was a chain-smoker; she was very irritable and seemed angry. We thought that perhaps she had quarrelled with the man she was sitting with. They seemed annoyed with each other and appeared to be silently expressing their anger.

At the time we didn't fully understand the meaning of my experience, but it did serve as a valuable lesson for me to be more aware of my own ability to see and feel auras. I now believe that the intake and influence of regular drugs do in fact hinder the quality of the aura and can in time cause serious health disorders.

Since that particular experience I have frequently seen people's auras, especially when I am in a colour counselling or colour therapy/healing session. I should say that this is a natural ability which comes and goes without any conscious effort on my part.

When it does come I always try to interpret my experiences in relation to the circumstances at that time. Once I saw a woman at a meeting covered with a dirty dull GREEN around her breast and chest region. Little did I know at the time that she was suffering from cancer of the breasts. Quite often, when a client comes to me and I see the colours of their aura, I will see dull or pale colours around them. This often depicts the client's state at the time. If the colours are vibrant and glowing radiantly, then I know the client is feeling happy and positive about their condition or particular situation. This is usually also expressed by the client during the session.

I remember seeing a radiant glow of luminous VIOLETS and PINKS around Belinda's head and shoulders at the beginning of one of her colour counselling sessions. During her session Belinda said that she had for the first time in her life (after 48 years) felt what it meant to recognise her sense of self-worth. For years she had belittled herself and allowed others to manipulate her to suit their own situation and needs. For the first time she was able to say 'no' to a friend who had tended to use her. I could clearly see the difference in her being: she was radiating self-respect and dignity, both of which are qualities associated with the colour VIOLET and this was the first colour chosen in her CRR.

Helen

When Helen came to see me for a colour therapy treatment, she was like a time-bomb ready to explode. Her aura was filled with bright RED, especially over the reproductive, base chakra and over the chest region. My immediate sense of Helen was that she had suffered some physical abuse, perhaps sexual, and was struggling to come to terms with her anger about this. Emotionally she was very closed and tense. Helen had a strong personality that could easily intimidate people and cause them to feel uncomfortable in her presence. During the session it seemed that 'she knew the answers to everything'. She tended to be very aggressive, domi-nant and extremely defensive. For a while I allowed this to con-tinue to see how far she would go, and then I became quite firm with her by saying that if she knew so much then why was she here? It seemed the most logical question to ask. I continued to say that if she continued with such an uncooperative attitude it would be impossible to help her and no doubt she would find it very difficult to find a therapist who would be willing to work with her under such stressful conditions. Suddenly she burst into tears and immediately I saw her aura colours change from bright RED in her chest to a lovely soft PINK as she became more gentle. This was the beginning of a long relationship between us and one that proved meaningful and challenging to us both.

The Chakra System

There are eight major centres within each level of the aura which absorb colour vibrations and circulate them round the complete system. These are the centres of power, known as the 'chakras' (from a Sanskrit word meaning Wheel of Fire). They form part of the auric body including the physical body, and they are all constantly moving, continuously absorbing specific currents of energy. A free flow of this energy is vital to the health and well-being of a person.

All the chakras interpenetrate one another, and are joined within the body at intervals along the spine. Each of the eight chakras correspond with a particular colour frequency, and with a particular gland or part of the human body. These glands are known as the endocrine glands and are constantly transmuting chemical elements into hormones to be carried through the bloodstream, each performing a different function (see Fig. 9).

The chakras work to attract a dominant energy vibration, which can help to restore health (physically, emotionally and mentally) and to maintain health in cases where disease has caused blockage or resistance. Imbalances of this kind suggest that there may be too much, or too little, of a particular colour energy in evidence, and this can happen for a number of reasons. In a healthy body, the chakras absorb and distribute energy evenly; in an unhealthy state, toxins may begin to collect which can eventually cause actual physical, emotional and/or mental problems.

The following details can be used in addition to the information given in Chapter 2 – The Super Eight Colours – to help you interpret the colours you have chosen from the Colour Reflection

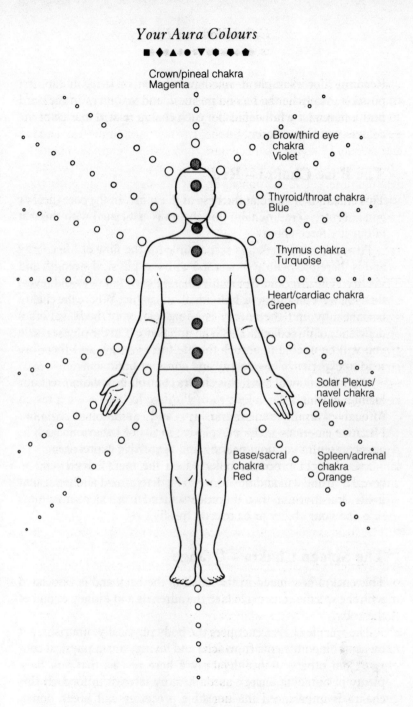

Crown/pineal chakra
Magenta

Brow/third eye
chakra
Violet

Thyroid/throat chakra
Blue

Thymus chakra
Turquoise

Heart/cardiac chakra
Green

Solar Plexus/
navel chakra
Yellow

Base/sacral
chakra
Red

Spleen/adrenal
chakra
Orange

Fig. 9 The Chakra System

Reading. For example if you have chosen ORANGE in the first position, GREEN in the second position, and MAGENTA in the third position, read the full details for each chakra related to each of the colours you have chosen.

The Base Chakra – Red

This chakra is situated at the base of the spine, in the coccygeal or gonad centre. Traditionally this chakra is associated with the seat of our life-force energy.

Physically this chakra is responsible for the flow of life energy and is therefore mainly concerned with our physical strength and vitality. A healthy and vibrantly radiating RED chakra would reveal that you were an energetic individual, full of life. Where the chakra is unhealthy and the energy is being lost, your body suffers a deficiency of this colour. This is an imbalance. On the physical side you will be unable to absorb the life-force energy, and therefore tend to experience low energy and constant tiredness.

On the emotional level, this chakra controls how we express our feelings through the colour RED. Positive feelings are expressed through warmth and friendship, and uninhibited passion. Negative emotions include explosive forms of behaviour such as anger, resentment, domineering and aggressive expressions.

RED thought processes reflected on the mental level tend to reveal a strong will and the desire to be determined and persistent in life. Negative RED thought processes tend to reflect your ruthless side and your ability to be overtly 'pushy'.

The Spleen Chakra – Orange

This chakra is situated in the small of the back and is associated with the splenic centre, close to the adrenals and kidney region of the body.

The splenic chakra energises the body physically, nourishing it by absorbing nutrients from food and loving, warm physical contact from others. A healthy chakra here reveals that you have plenty of outgoing energy and a healthy interest in food. If this chakra is imbalanced the digestive processes will break down, preventing proper assimilation and distribution of food substances within your body and can often lead to a general loss of appetite, leading to tiredness and lack of vitality.

The emotional value of this chakra associated with the colour ORANGE is that it encourages joy, fun and pleasure. Positive qualities reflected on the emotional level reveal that you have courage and confidence, and are able to communicate and interact with others freely. Negative emotional expressions here reveal that you are fearful, timid and shy. A blocked splenic chakra suggests the inability to register and respond to external stimuli.

If you have a healthy ORANGE chakra your thought processes will show you have a happy interest in life and in your future potential. You will show a sense of excitement and enthusiasm to go forward, positively and constructively, and make the best of life's pleasures. Negative thought processes reveal a tendency to try too hard and thereby place yourself under tremendous strain, often resulting in mental dissipation.

The Solar Plexus Chakra – Yellow

The solar plexus chakra is situated between the naval and the rib cage. It relates to the autonomic nervous system as well as to the pancreas and the liver. It is the largest of all the chakras and is the most powerful. It deals with the purifying processes of the body, clearing out toxins in the digestive system, the adrenal glands, the pancreas and the liver.

The physical aspects of this chakra, related to the colour YELLOW, has a stimulating effect on the nerves. If this chakra is healthy and balanced you will radiate a sense of being in control and will physically have good co-ordination and orientation. If on the other hand it is imbalanced you will probably suffer from a nervous disorder or express sickness and loss of vitality and energy in the body generally.

The positive emotional aspects of this chakra reflect that you are powerful and an achiever. You will be warm-hearted, enjoying being the centre of attention and often boldly outspoken. The negative emotional aspects reveal you feel a lack of power and experience feelings of being disorientated and dissipated in life. You can become obsessional and may express many insecurities.

The mental aspects of the YELLOW chakra relate to our ability to grasp things well on the mental level. This chakra focuses on the intellectual powers and is attached to the development of our knowledge and the left hemisphere of the brain. Usually a lot of YELLOW on this level reveals interests or involvement in the scientific fields. With little YELLOW here it implies a lack of use of the mental faculties and that you have little belief in your mental capabilities. You will tend to get confused and frustrated if things don't go your own way.

The Heart Chakra – Green

The heart chakra is linked with the physical heart and with the blood circulation. The colour associated with this chakra is GREEN. It lies between the solar plexus chakra (YELLOW) and the thymus chakra (TURQUOISE).

On the physical level it is connected with the functioning of the heart, blood and the chest region as a whole. If this chakra is working well you will experience a life free from heart troubles and blood disorders. Problems to do with the heart, blood and chest region are connected with an imbalance in this centre. High/low blood pressure, heart murmurs, cancer and cysts etc. are such problems.

The expression of the heart centre on the emotional level reveals that you are understanding, co-operative and seek harmony and balance in life. GREEN on this level can express tendencies to be least concerned with personal desires and more concerned with sharing with others. A healthy expression of this chakra shows an appreciation for the simple things in life, that you value what you have, and feel contented. Negative expressions on the emotional level show that you are overly reserved, cautious and emotionally saddened, afraid to step out and fully participate in life.

The expression of the GREEN chakra on the mental level shows that you enjoy what life has to offer and are assured of a constant supply (of money, food, emotional support etc.), to help fulfil your needs. On the negative side the expression is to believe the opposite, that life is unfair and unjust and that the world tends to deal out harsh realities. You tend to see yourself as a helpless victim of society.

The Thymus Chakra – Turquoise

This chakra is situated between the heart chakra (GREEN) and the thyroid chakra (BLUE), midway between the shoulder blades. This organ has not been given the recognition from the medical profession that it truly deserves. Perhaps this is because as we grow older it diminishes in size to a point where it is hardly recognisable. However since 1960 the thymus gland has been associated with the production of a hormone (thymosin), which has been shown to have a direct effect on the immunological system. The thymus is therefore a vital organ which helps to produce antibodies and therefore to prevent foreign bodies and bacteria entering the physical system. An unhealthy thymus chakra will be unable to prevent disease in the body and therefore the immune system will be weakened resulting in the breakdown of our defence system.

The emotional expression of this chakra related to the colour TURQUOISE on the positive side, reveals that you are well-adjusted and capable of interacting with people socially. You will bring a new and refreshing energy to ordinary, everyday situations. Another quality on the positive side allows you to enjoy your own company, while on the negative side you may tend to 'enjoy' emotional trauma and require long periods of retreat and have the need to be alone, disconnecting from colleagues, friends and/or family. Onlookers may see this as an expression of childish sulking, and one of immature behaviour.

Mentally the expression of the TURQUOISE chakra is to be very positive, looking ahead into the future and seeing only good things. The thought processes here are optimistic and tend to see things clearly. You will usually show a willingness to try new 'alternatives' and are prepared to learn from past mistakes. Negative mental expressions reveal much confusion, turmoil and the inability to move through your own boundaries and limitations. Ultimately this can lead to negative self-destructive thought-forms about the Self and of others.

The Thyroid Chakra – Blue

This chakra is situated at the front of the base of the neck. It is linked with the thyroid and the parathyroid glands, which are concerned with the important role of controlling the metabolic rate and balances body equilibrium.

The physical expression of this chakra when it is working properly is to regulate our ability to express ourselves vocally. It is associated with the medium of sound and has a lot to do with our vocal expression and verbal communication. A physically over-active thyroid reveals that you are using up a great deal of energy and as a result get tired very easily and have the tendency to fatigue quickly, while an underactive thyroid reveals that you tend to be sluggish and slow in your bodily movements and tend to experience many sore throat problems and colds as a result.

Emotional expression of this chakra shows that you are sensitive and often able to hear sounds from other dimensions, i.e. other than the physical. This is where the ability to experience clair-audience takes place. If you are involved with using the creative expression of the voice, as a singer or even a public speaker, you may tend to have a larger thyroid centre than most, because of its regular use. A negative expression here would reveal that you find it difficult to express yourself and therefore tend to keep rather quiet, subdued and generally withdrawn from others.

The mental and positive expressions of the BLUE chakra suggests that you are spiritually aware and are interested in the more finer qualities of life. You believe in taking time to be alone with your own thoughts to reflect, contemplate and meditate about life in general. Often you tend to philosophise about the purpose of human existence and seek to explore or discover your inner nature. On the negative side your thought processes tend to be involved in areas that may have little or no relevance to everyday life situations. You may have difficulty in motivating yourself and in putting things into practice.

The Brow/Third Eye Chakra – Violet

This chakra is associated with the pituitary gland and is situated at the base of the brain. It governs the hormones of the other endo-crine glands and plays a major role in the normal functioning of the physical body as a whole. When functioning properly this gland aids sleep, and purifies the body. It helps to relieve many disorders including neuralgia, kidney problems and nervousness. In general it calms and soothes the mind and influences the organs of sight, hearing and smelling and thus is used effectively to relieve problems in the eyes, ears and nose.

The emotional expression of this chakra is connected with our sense of self-respect and pride. You would express a powerful ability to capture people's attention, and, when this chakra is operating normally, you are capable of connecting with your spiritual/psychic abilities which include clairvoyancy and telepathy. When the chakra is operating negatively, however, you tend to feel low self-worth and generally unappreciated by others. You see yourself as being inferior to others and often become paranoid about yourself in the company of others.

The mental expression of this chakra reflects that your thinking is often abstract and with a tendency to be futuristic. You may be a visionary, with ideas and ideals many years ahead of your time. You receive inspiration from subtle planes and intangible sources and with it come images and impressions in the form of symbols, which usually need to be translated into more tangible expressions. The negative expression on the mental level is to experience fears and phobias, and to rely heavily on the intellect, not trusting your intuition, and constantly doubting and apologising for yourself.

The Crown Chakra – Magenta

The MAGENTA chakra is located at the top of the head and is associated with the function of the brain and the pineal gland. It is interconnected with all the other chakras, and therefore any imbalance in the crown chakra is reflected in most of the other centres as well.

The physical expression of the pineal gland has been found to be intrinsically linked with the hormone melatonin, the substance which pigments our skin. The pineal gland also produces hormones which control other biological functions and has several endocrine connections. If this chakra shows signs of an imbalance, the physical disorders may result in problems connected to the sympathetic nervous system, both minor and severe forms of headaches and migraine problems, and others related to the brain and the scalp.

The emotional expression of the MAGENTA crown chakra on the

positive side allow you to show much love and compassion towards others, and to feel a sense of affection, kindness and gentleness towards your fellow human beings. On the negative emotional side of this chakra you can be domineering, forceful and threatening, and may tend to behave arrogantly under the guise of 'love' and 'spirituality'. A further emotional expression related to an imbalanced MAGENTA chakra is for you to deny your needs to the point of self-sacrifice and martyrdom.

The positive and mental expression of the MAGENTA chakra tend to be related to your spiritual quality and the state of your consciousness and level of maturity. It reflects your inner strength. Your thought processes tend to be concerned with other people's needs rather than your own. You tend to be wise and knowledgeable in many aspects of life and to see the positive side of things rather than the negative. On the negative side, you may believe that you are inferior to others, and try to be in control of situations and even people. This side of the MAGENTA mental chakra tends to make it very difficult for you to admit to your own faults and failings, which ultimately means it is difficult for you to let go of situations you have initiated.

Balancing the Chakras

Where there are depletions or excesses of any colour energy within the chakras, balance and replenishment can be achieved by re-introducing the appropriate colour into one's life, and in this book we outline methods to help you achieve this. One practical example would be in the case of a sore throat or cough. Here we suggest that the colour BLUE needs to be introduced regularly, to assist in strengthening the thyroid chakra and its associated part of the body, the throat and the back of the neck. By using the colour breathing, colour visualisation and colour affirmation exercises described in Chapter 7 you can reduce and even relieve pain and discomfort within your system. You can also work with particular emotional or mental areas you feel need improving.

chapter 4

■ ◆ ▲ ● ▼ ◈ ■ ⬠

THE HISTORY OF COLOUR

Symbolic Colour

Colour and light have always been an essential part of life and our existence of Earth. One of the earliest records of the magical powers of colour can be seen in the grottos of Lascaux and Altimara, where decorative paintings of various animals adorn the interior cave walls. Painted by hand using the simplest, natural pigments available from the cave floor, RED and YELLOW ochre, BLACK manganese and mud, a considerable variety of colours have been found in cave art. In Lascaux and Altimara the calcite crystals that sparkle and line the caves walls introduced WHITE into the paintings to create and produce subtle shades and effective perspectives.

Prehistoric man soon realised the importance of colour with the changes of colours in nature: the cycle of day into night,when the sun set a RED dusk indicated the end of daily activity and the need to withdraw into the safety of the caves to avoid the possible dangers of the dark, BLACK night. RED and BLACK are the colours symbolic of life and death. They were first used by Neanderthal Man to decorate the graves of his dead and later the same colours were used by his successors to adorn their first works of art.

As mankind developed, the expression of his works of art shifted from cave paintings and wall decoration to self-decoration and body painting, found among tribal communities. This could be seen at first from the use of various natural materials such as leaves, feathers, shells and coloured paint. Within each tribe and community all members adorned the surface of their body with their own BLUE-print to express their particular relation to society. This usually occurred at those crucial times in life when an individual passed from one status to another, e.g. at birth, puberty, marriage and death.

Body painting and self-decoration showed one's membership in and identification with a particular community and designated status within that community, as well as defining social roles. Particular colours and styles allowed members of a tribe and of other tribes to recognise each other and so it acted as a form of clothing, just as policemen wear BLACK uniforms, businessmen wear BLUE suits, nurses and doctors wear WHITE coats.

Today body painting takes many forms. People adorn themselves with a variety of coloured make-up, usually on the face. Women wear make-up to alter the shape and appearance of their features, enhancing their natural colouring at the same time and performers use it to create the best and most striking effects under the strongest of lighting.

The Egyptians synthesised a BLUE pigment (most likely as a result of glass-making experiments) to symbolise divinity, truth and integrity. These were colour attributes which were later to re-emerge in the cloaked Madonna of Christian symbolism. Even today in British marriages the colour BLUE is familiar to everyone. The rhyme 'Something old and something new, something borrowed and something BLUE' holds the same deep meaningful associations similar to that considered by the ancient Egyptians.

In India a Hindu bride wore old YELLOW clothing for six days before her wedding in order to drive away evil spirits. At the wedding ceremony she wore YELLOW, as did the priest who conducted the ceremony, while in China the bride-to-be wore RED, symbolic of new life, good fortune and happiness for the future. WHITE was the basic colour of the Greek Parthenon (meaning 'virginity') and of Athena's statue, and is still the most popularly displayed colour worn by Western brides.

TYRIAN PURPLE was the most sacred colour for the Greeks and Romans. Extracted from the mures, a kind of whelk, it was the colour reserved for the robes adorned by gods and emperors. This was probably because of the expense involved to produce it.

Colour in Sacred Buildings and Religion

The 'Mountain of God' at Ur (now in Iraq), a tower unearthed by
Leonard Woollery in the 1920s, is recognised as one of the oldest
buildings in the world, dating back to 230 BC. The colours of its
four concentric walls are BLACK and RED, topped with BLUE and
GOLD.

The walls of the ancient Chinese capital Peking were painted
RED and roofs within the city were coloured YELLOW to symbolise
good and evil spirits. The interiors of the ancient Egyptians'
temples often contained BLUE painted ceilings to symbolise the
heavens, while GREEN was used on the floors to represent the
meadows of the Nile.

The Greeks used colour to intensify form and shape. Various
tones of BLUE were applied to underline the shadows on
limewashed Ionian capitals and RED columns of Knossos were used
to emphasise the weight and heaviness borne by the supports,
giving sharp contrast to the BLUE Mediterranean sky above and the
sea below.

Even today, on the many islands of Greece, doors and window
shutters are frequently painted in TURQUOISE and BLUE. WHITE is
used to reflect the heat of the sun (which is common to most hot
countries, because WHITE reflects the heat and gives the sensation
of feeling cool), and TURQUOISE and BLUE blend in with the
Mediterranean sea and sky.

It was the use of pigment processing in pottery glazing and
glass-making which helped to advance and extend this medium.
The production of glass gave colour a luminosity beautifully
exploited in Greek, Roman and Byzantine mosaics and later in
stained-glass windows in medieval cathedrals, allowing a complete
spectral display of coloured light to pour on to the surfaces of their
interiors. Many French churches still show the distinguishable
colours on their exterior walls, flecks of RED, BLUE and GREEN at
Angers and the RED stain on Notre Dame.

Further east is Cyprus where some of the world's most famous
and intact mosaics exist, you can see an array of REDS, YELLOWS,
BLUES and GREENS on the wall and floor mosaic displays, depicting
scenes of important events that took place in the region.

The colour in the clothes worn by gods and goddesses, priests and emperors etc. all had religious significance. In Egypt the colours associated with the Sun God Ra were GOLD, RED and YELLOW, and in Greece GOLD was assigned to Athena, who wore a GOLDEN robe. The RED poppy was sacred to Ceres, goddess of the harvest, while the colour PURPLE was worn by Ulysses to signify his sea odyssey. VIOLET, the colour worn by the monarch, was reserved for the dressing of the altar and lectern to match the vestments worn by priests in the Greek and Russian Orthodox religion, as well as the Roman Catholic Church and the Church of England.

In the Orient the Hindu religion Brahmanism is recognised by the colours of YELLOW and GOLD which were considered sacred. The Buddha wore tunics of GOLD and YELLOW in praise of the higher spiritual wisdom but wore RED when pondering over the changing fortune of man. Confucius was also identified with YELLOW, but not with PURPLE, because he felt it confused him with RED. In fact Confucius showed a great dislike for this colour and expressed this in his writings. According to the book *Heang Tang*, he wrote, 'The superior man did not use a deep PURPLE or a puce colour in the ornament of his dress.'

Colour in Healing

Ancient and Traditional Methods

Colour healing was widely practised by the ancient Egyptians, Babylonians and Assyrians in the art of Heliotherapy. They recognised the powerful therapeutic affects of the sun's rays and regularly exposed their bodies to it for healing purposes. They also recognised the significance of light and colour rays contained within crystals and gemstones found within the Earth's crust. For exemple, gemstones, crystals and precious stones were used as forms of transmitters to promote healing. These natural stones and crystals were considered to be filled with coloured light and energy which could be used to relieve different types of ailments. By grounding and crushing, diluting and or dipping them in water, they were considered to be imbued with a strange, mystical quality, enabling them to be used as a remedy for the sick. In certain parts of the world, medicines have been mixed with crushed gold and pearls for rheumatism, bronchitis and epilepsy; emeralds for diabetes; rubies for the heart and brain. Turquoise was used for protection against poison, for example bites from reptiles. Amber was mixed with honey for eye problems and earaches, and carnelian was thought to restrain haemorrhage and relieve sores and blotchiness from the skin. Jade was said to assist in pregnancy and lapis lazuli was meant to prevent miscarriage. In recent times there has been a huge revival of interest in crystal healing, and colour visualisation is a vital element in its practice.

It was probably not until the time of the Greek clinician that much thought was given to the physical rather than the metaphysical nature of colour. Hippocrates attempted to take a more practical and scientific medical point of view. As the 'Father of Medicine', he founded the diagnostic approach on which modern-day medicine is based and developed a method known as the Doctrine of the Humours. Each of the four humours (which related to the four elements, Fire, Earth, Air, Water) had its associated colour, and ill-health was seen by diagnosing the condition of a patient according to the colour variations of the hair, skin and eyes, as well as the colour of excrement and urine.

To this day the observation of the coloration of the skin, tongue and eyes and the secretions of the body act as the basis of diagnosis throughout the world.

Celsus who lived at the beginning of the Christian era believed that placing coloured plasters over the wounds of patients would help the healing process, particularly if the plasters were of the same colour as that of the illness itself, e.g. a RED plaster would rapidly cicatrise a wound. This idea seems similar to one of the principles of homeopathy, the practice of treating like with like. He also applied various herbs and oils: WHITE and PURPLE violets, lily, rose and saffron were given, based on the value of their colours. Saffron ointment and iris-oil were applied on the head to help calm the mind and induce sleep.

Galen, the famous Greco-Roman physician, AD 130–200, felt motion and change were important factors in diagnosis, and developed a theory where visible colour changes were addressed; for example, if 'that which is WHITE becomes BLACK, or that which is BLACK becomes WHITE it undergoes motion in respect to colour'.

The changes of the visible colours of an imbalance could indicate the different stages through which the imbalance moved. The first appearance of a bruise begins with a RED patch on the skin. Then it develops by turning deep BLACK and BLUE. After a few days the bruise changes colour to dark PURPLE, then alters to GREEN and eventually YELLOWISH until the bruise fades away completely.

The Arabian physician, Avicenna (980–1039), whose *Canon of Medicine* was one of the most remarkable medical documentations ever about colour both as a guide in diagnosis and also as an actual curative, studied the strength of a person's breathing patterns and associated these with the elements and their associated colours. For example the breath of Earth was slow, while the breath of Fire was quick. Extending Hippocrates' doctrine of the humours, he believed that innate temperament might be found within hair colour: People with black hair had hot temperaments and people with brown hair had cold temperaments. People suffering from nose-bleeding should avoid RED and those with eye defects should avoid RED and YELLOW. He found that BLUE had a soothing effect upon the movement of the blood, while RED stimulated it.

The Chinese still apply colour for diagnostic purposes by observing and checking the coloration or discoloration of different parts of the body, one of the most effective ways of assessing the state of health of a patient. The body is divided into twelve different regions, each of which can be diagnosed as healthy or unhealthy, according to its colour. For example, REDNESS in the eyes signifies conjunctivitis; bloodshot lines with dots on the end are signs of hardening and stagnation in the blood circulation. The colour of the eyeball is related to the liver and the pupil is related to kidney problems. The WHITES of the eye relate to the lungs and the upper and lower lids of the eye relate to the stomach. Similarly the colour of the nails reveals among other things the condition of the liver. The variations of colour of the urine, stools, skin, hair, lips, tongue, pulse-rate, ears, complexion as well as the general and overall appearance of the individual, in terms of posture, motion, tone of voice, and the emotional state, are all taken into account. Examples of different coloured pulse-rates are as follows: a fast pulse-rate (RED) would indicate heat and overactivity in the body, while a GREEN pulse-rate warns of sluggishness or congestion.

The Hindus use solarised water, a system of placing different coloured containers filled with water and placed in the path of direct sunlight and later given to the patient to drink. This was meant to relieve the aches and pains of those who were ill. Of course the traditional form of working with colour for the Hindus is with the chakra system, described in the previous chapter.

Modern Treatments

With the development of modern methods of therapeutic treatment, and of surgery and medicines generally, colour therapy was not considered a form of medicine worthy of serious research and investigation. However, Edwin D. Babbitt (1828–1905), a writer on humanism and a professor at Harvard, spent many years writing *The Principles of Colour and Light* (1878). Mainly through his efforts (and those of his near contemporary Pancoast), interest in the field of ethereal planes of energy and the powers of light and colour were revived. A variation on the traditional occult practice of alchemy was adopted, employing colour in relation to elements and minerals and a system of 'thermal', 'luminous' and 'electrical' colours. By 'thermal', Babbitt meant the warm colours RED and ORANGE which he considered to radiate heat and warmth. 'Electrical' described the BLUE range colours – i.e. BLUE and VIOLET – which were cold in principle. 'Luminosity' expressed the brightness of yellow, the colour closest to the sun.

RED light, a thermal colour, was especially good for rousing effects upon the blood and to some extent upon the nerves. It helped particularly in cases where patients suffered from paralysis. YELLOW and ORANGE stimulated the nerves, and YELLOW excited the brain. BLUE and VIOLET were calming and soothing colours, useful in relaxing and reducing inflammatory conditions such as sciatica, headaches, sunstroke and nervous irritability.

Babbitt's colour treatment employed a range of instruments so that the patient could be bathed with coloured light. The Thermo-lume, for instance, used natural sunlight directed through stained-glass filters and absorbed by the patient who would be sitting in a chair behind.

He worked with the three primaries: RED as the centre of heat, the ruling spectrum of hydrogen (a heat-producing colour); YELLOW, the centre of luminosity; and BLUE the centre of electricity, the ruling spectrum of oxygen. In colour therapy it is necessary to have unity and affinity, balance and harmony. Therefore he felt it necessary to use colours in contrast to and in harmony with each other. Any one colour had its complementary, for example RED and BLUE, YELLOW and VIOLET etc.

During Babbitt's time many colour-therapy practices were opened and established throughout the world. The second edition of this book brought him international recognition and fame, although his works were frequently criticised by the American Medical Association. Generally speaking, doctors and scientists regarded the use of colour for healing purposes with scepticism, even though they used the invisible power of light (infrared and ultraviolet light and X-rays are now proven methods of treating growths, tumours, skin tanning, the destruction of bacteria, etc.).

Rudolf Steiner (1861–1925) a researcher of spiritual, scientific and religious teachings, spent over forty years studying the nature of colour. As a child he experienced the reality of the spiritual aspects of the world, which he sought to harmonise with the findings of science. Later Steiner was invited to edit Goethe's scientific work, which helped him to achieve this integration. In his book *Theosophy and Knowledge of the Higher Worlds* he began to describe the auric colours as they are seen with spiritual perception.

In his lectures Steiner showed his listeners how to look at colour in a way that raised not only the theory but also practical technique into the realm of art. Steiner developed Goethe's theory on the laws and subtleties of colour and form metamorphosis. He developed a new artistic style employing form and colour, and pioneered eurythmy, a new art form of movement in which every gesture is either light or dark, and every mood is felt to be coloured.

In his painting technique he observed the different colour qualities in the kingdoms of mineral, plant, animal and man. He also introduced the distinction between image and lustre colours, both completely new concepts in the theory of colour. In 1913 he founded the Anthroposophical Society.

In the early to mid part of this century, Dr Roland Hunt produced several books which described the uses of colour for diagnostic and treatment purposes. Hunt researched the effects of colour in relation to sound and music, perfume and lighting, and developed a complete range of colour lamps and lighting equipment for use in our objective environment. These he saw could act as a key or doorway through which higher forms of colour healing could operate subjectively. His lamps were also designed with therapeutic quality in mind, as well as for aesthetic beauty, which he felt served to raise and uplift human consciousness.

Theophilus Gimbel, a Bavarian by birth now living in Britain, is one of the most respected colour therapists of this century. He too has developed various colour illumination instruments to project coloured light for healing purposes, many of his ideas being based on the work of Goethe, Steiner, Babbitt and Hunt.

Gimbel has developed a similar colour illumination instrument or cabinet to that of Babbitt's 'Thermolume', but instead of using natural sunlight to pass through the stained-glass filters to be projected on to the patient, he replaced the sunlight with artificial electric light. He also applied the principles of Goethe's work which brought forward the ideas of using complementarities, and the concept that colours were created by the interplay of light and dark.

As a colour therapist practising for over thirty years, Theophilus Gimbel has done much to further the work of colour therapy and initiate more investigations into this field. To him we owe much, as it was with him that we began our initial study into this fascinating subject. Some of the basic ideas we use in our work have been influenced by him and his predecessors. Together, their teachings have helped to develop our own system.

Living Colour and the Colour Reflection Reading

With the development and increasing awareness in the field of psychosomatic medicine, our work with colour therapy found greater meaning. Unless our fears and tensions are able to be expressed, relieved and understood, the physiological and biological elements of our being cannot be healed. To deny the importance of man's psyche and its connection with the physical body would be similar to treating the symptoms of the disease rather than dealing with the entire organism. For example, to treat a person suffering from severe headaches or migraine, allergies or stress; not only the physical problem but also the metaphysical factors that helped to create the problem in the first place must be taken into account.

By developing the Colour Reflection Reading we were able to offer a powerful and effective entry point into these realms. In order to take the CRR one stage further, the client can experience colour therapy treatment, using the concept of complementary colours alongside crystals. The instrument used here – The Colour-Light-Crystal Unit, is based on the original design developed by Godfrey Thomas, a former dentist and a dear friend. This instrument offers a new dimension to the experience of colour therapy, which gives the sensation that the colours are more vibrant and 'alive'. Students and clients have responded positively towards the instrument and enjoy the variety and depth it offers. We have now developed the instrument further and use it at our clinic as one of the ways of experiencing colour therapy treatment.

We believe that the use of colour therapy is intrinsically linked with the human body physiologically and psychologically. The healing of diseases deals as much with the emotions, the mind and the spirit of man as with the body itself. This is why we also place great importance in our Colour Counselling Service. We feel that being aware of one's problems is the first step to overcoming them, and unless the individual is willing to move through them and take action to change their attitude or life-style accordingly, the problem will remain.

Colour counselling is an essential part of colour therapy treatment and should be recognised for its long-term benefits which help people to see things more objectively and go forward with more confidence and self-esteem. We talk more about our work in Chapter 8.

chapter 5

■ ◆ ▲ ● ▼ ◆ ⬠

COLOUR FOR CLOTHES

Clothes allow you to express yourself through your choice of colour. Knowing yourself better through the Colour Reflection Reading and understanding your overall 'colour state' acts as a powerful and positive expression of who you are. Instead of haphazardly experimenting with colour for the sake of it, or projecting yourself in a 'manufactured' way, with a little knowledge of colour, you can balance your inner and outer state as a whole.

With modern technology and advanced methods of making literally thousands of colours, it is easy for us to become 'colour polluted', 'colour confused' or even 'colour crazy' when there are so many and different types of colours – such as 'day-glo' colours and other strong synthetic colours – on the market. Colour for its own sake leaves us feeling disorientated and out of touch with ourselves, becoming merely a tool to cover up, hide, manipulate or stimulate attention for the wrong reasons. Colour can, on the other hand, be used productively and constructively.

In this section we present four sets of colours and explain how you can be associated with one of these categories. Once you know which category you belong to, you can experiment and play, becoming more colour conscious in dress.

Clothes are like colour filters over our bodies which regulate and determine the quantity and quality of colour and light energy that is absorbed in our physical and subtle body. This colour and energy will eventually affect us and we need to consider carefully what we wear in order to be able to live in balance and harmony.

The colours people wear reveal a lot about them. The next time you are on a train or a bus, or walking in the street, look around and make a mental note of the colours people wear. What do you notice? Then choose a particular individual and see what their colour image reveals.

The following section will give you some guidelines as to the statements people make about themselves simply by the colours they choose to wear in their clothes.

Psychological Effects of Colour in Clothes

Red This colour makes you feel more energetic, outgoing and ready to move forward in some overt way. It tends to catch people's eye and attract attention. If you wear RED you may wish to be seen as having fire and passion, ferocity and strength. Those who like action and drama like to wear this colour. Wearing RED can also denote a strong sexuality.

Orange An energetic and stimulating colour, it doesn't have quite the same 'push' as RED. If you're fond of wearing ORANGE you may have a courageous and adventurous streak, showing enthusiasm and zeal in whatever you do, even if it draws on your energy. People who wear this colour are assertive and like to smile and make others smile. Wearing ORANGE also encourages conversation and a sense of humour.

Yellow This colour is often worn by intellectuals, the studious and those who like to be in positions of authority and control. It encourages open-mindedness and attention to detail. Wearing YELLOW 'brings in the light'. It is the colour mostly associated with the sun and tends to generate positive and optimistic qualities in those who wear it.

Green This colour helps people to create calm, soothing and balancing atmospheres around them. It stands for harmony and equilibrium. GREEN in clothes tends to reflect the conventional types, those who like to stick to the straight and narrow and who perfer not to stand out in a crowd. Those who like this colour usually appreciate nature and the security it brings.

Turquoise   This colour encourages people to show an interest in you. It stimulates a quiet refreshing personality who is easily approachable. It helps you to be clear in your thoughts and your feelings, generating clarity in your communication. If you like to wear TURQUOISE you may wish to be seen as having youthfulness and sparkle.

Blue   Wearing BLUE suggests spirituality and order. Those who wear it reflect a wish for peace and quiet, tranquillity and even solitude. It is a non-threatening colour and the individual who wears it probably values loyalty and honesty.

Violet   Wearing VIOLET generates feelings of self-respect, dignity and self-worth. It is a colour worn by Catholic priests to reflect sanctity and humility. Because of its richness, it is also associated with the monarch, extravagance and wealth. Many artists favour this colour in clothes, perhaps because of its creative or spiritual qualities.

Magenta   Wearing this colour generates feelings of softness, gentleness and kindness. It creates affection and feelings of love and compassion. Because of the RED contribution to creating this colour it also generates a powerful sexual message, which can be subtly manipulative. If you like wearing this colour it could be because you wish to express your sensuality.

Black   In most Western societies BLACK is almost universally the colour of death, grief and penitence. It is often worn by those who reject society or rebel against the norm within society. It is a colour which denies the light and those who wear it reject the light in themselves, by pushing it away and not allowing it to be absorbed. It is the colour worn by businessmen, policemen and priests to reflect power and authority. BLACK is accepted as being dark and mysterious and has also come to mean sexy. Yet BLACK is also for those who like to appear traditional and respectable.

White   In clothes WHITE has been associated with cleanliness, purity and innocence. In the East WHITE is worn as the colour appropriate for death and mourning, accepting that the deceased has departed the physical world for the purer, spiritual one. WHITE is the colour of detachment. WHITE reflects all colour and those who wear it may do so to keep themselves cool in the heat of the sun's rays.

Brown   The colour BROWN is often associated with the earth and with stability. To create BROWN you need the colour RED mixed with BLACK, therefore it has many of their attributes. BROWN is a colour concerned with groundedness and building firm foundations for the future (similar to that of positive RED). It also contains the powerful quality of BLACK in that it relates to authority, inner confidence and self-assuredness. A person who likes to wear BROWN is likely to be highly dedicated and committed to their work, family and friends. On the positive side, they are practical and materialistic in life, but on the negative they can be deeply insecure and unstable. The colour BROWN generates being organised and steadfast, especially in day-to-day responsibilities. Those who like the colour BROWN are able to get to the 'root' of things and deal with complicated matters simply and directly. They are 'no nonsense' people.

A further note on BLACK

BLACK is the absorption or the denial of all colour. Often we use the phrase 'BLACK mood' which suggest feeling unhappy, withdrawn, depressed, miserable. It is also associated with death and the unknown, the dark or shadow side of the self. It is an excellent colour for hiding oneself or covering an item to blend into the background.

We often feel sad to see so many people in the streets, and of course those who come to our clinic, wearing only BLACK. It takes such little effort to include just a small amount of colour, especially when there are such beautiful colours available. Many clients have come to receive colour therapy wearing all BLACK from head to toe, and usually our response to this is to find out if wearing BLACK is a colour they wear a lot or if this is just a one-off. Those who wear it often will probably agree that they tend to feel inhibited in their expression of life and sit on the edges of situations looking in, rather than actively participating. They tend to be suppressed, especially on the emotional level.

Colour for Clothes

■ ◆ ▲ ● ▼ ● ● ♠

However the people we meet who wear a lot of BLACK, and who receive colour therapy treatment, find they soon become disinterested with all the BLACK around them as they begin to experience more zest for life. They try to bring at least one of the spectral hues into their dress, to bring out the colour rather than to emphasise the darkness of BLACK.

For some people the change-over is a gradual one; for others it is very quick and dramatic. Some find it difficult to let go of the safety net and security that BLACK provides, which reflects an unwillingness to discover more about their unconscious self.

A black case history

Liz first came to us in 1985 suffering from manic depression. She had experienced approximately 14 years of depression and had been to see several psychotherapists without much success. On arrival, we quickly noticed that she wore a long BLACK woollen coat, BLACK velvet ski-pants, BLACK boots and a BLACK V-neck jumper. She had a pale, sallow complexion, BROWN-GREEN eyes which were heavily made-up with BLACK kohl pencil, and brown hair. Liz was 47 years old. She had trained as an interior designer, but had not worked professionally for about seven years. When we asked her to choose three colours from the CRR she asked why BLACK or WHITE were not included. We replied that we concentrated on the spectrum colours only and considered BLACK and WHITE to be extreme colours from which the spectrum colours we use are created. This seemed to satisfy her, but we felt she was disappointed that BLACK was not on the agenda. When we asked her whether, had BLACK and WHITE been included in our selection process would she have chosen one of them, she said that she would probably have chosen BLACK first. Instead she chose BLUE first, ORANGE second and VIOLET third.

For five months Liz wore black despite the recommendation we gave her to wear ORANGE as the colour most beneficial to her condition. Then one day she arrived wearing a stunning autumnal ORANGE skirt, with a golden YELLOW blouse and a wide satin, ORANGE belt. The only BLACK in sight were her BLACK boots and BLACK coat. This was the first overt sign that the therapy was making an impact on her. When asked what caused her to change like this she said she wasn't quite sure, but simply on waking one

— 95 —

morning, she had just felt like wearing ORANGE. She had received many colour therapy treatments where she was bathed with ORANGE light, complemented with BLUE. This, we believe, had an accumulative effect on her aura, as well as the supportive colour visualisation and colour breathing techniques which we had taught her to use at any time she felt low.

Colour for Dress

Colour is an essential feature of the way we dress, and should be a natural expression of our personality. When it relates to our own natural colouring we feel more confident and self-assured than when there is a clash.

If you want to wear colours which will complement your natural colouring, you need first to take a look at the colour of your eyes, hair and skin. Wearing the wrong colours tends to attract attention to the colours themselves and detract from your general aesthetic harmony. 'Wrong' colours also tend to emphasise skin blemishes, lines and wrinkles. Patchy WHITE skin and RED blotches are actually enhanced by the wrong colours and they can make a person look older. The whites of the eyes look dull, and seem to lose their natural sparkle. The 'wrong' colours also give people a tired, drained and depleted look and a messy appearance. That's what we mean by expressions such as 'off colour' and 'washed out'.

The correct colours, on the other hand, will immediately reduce or minimise skin blemishes. The skin will look smoother, clearer, fresher and more alive. The eyes will sparkle, look bigger and seem brighter. The correct colours will enhance and bring out your own natural colouring, blending and harmonising not only with your skin tone, but also with your eyes and hair.

The principle of finding your 'true' colours is based on the work of the colour theorist Johannes Itten. Itten, an artist and a teacher at the Bauhaus School of Art in Germany, explored various methods of contrasting and combining colour, and found that many of his students were using colours in their work which harmonised exactly with their own personal colouring. Some would choose colours that were clear, crisp and sharp, while others always preferred muted, dusky shades of the same colours. Itten observed that students with dark hair and dark skin chose sharp colours such as BLACK, GREY, NAVY and BLUE. His theory used the three primary colours: RED, BLUE and YELLOW. All other inter-mediate colours could be produced from these with the use of BLACK and WHITE.

A system was then developed in America which divides people into four basic groups, each named after a season of the year. These seasons can then be subdivided into two parts, containing the cool spectrum colours, and the warm spectrum colours. Winter and Summer are classified as 'cool' because the underlying tone in their colours is BLUE-based. Spring and Autumn are classified as 'warm' seasons, becaue the underlying tone in their colours is YELLOW/GOLD.

If your natural colouring is enhanced by wearing the cool spectrum colours you are a Winter or a Summer person. If your natural colouring needs the warm spectrum colours you are a Spring or Autumn person.

Within the seasons themselves, Winter and Spring include the clearer colours, while Autumn and Summer tend to be more muted. Yet Autumn contains some clear colours as well. The process of choosing your season must take place in daylight or in artificial light which reproduces the same colour temperature (see p. 166).

The procedure normally then involves the use of special coloured fabrics, which are draped across you in turn, and observed both for intensity and clarity, in relation to your own natural colouring.

The next section gives you more information to help you determine your own season and discover the colours which suit you best. On p. 110, you will find out how to introduce colours that relate to the Colour Reflection Reading.

Determining Your Colouring

To determine your season and the colours that are best suited to you, you need to take a good look at your skin (without make-up, if you use it); eyes and hair are important factors as well. You should also read the section beginning on p. 101 on Personality, Colour and the Seasons, to check that your personality traits correspond with the season you think you are.

The three pigments that determine the colour of your skin are melanin (BROWN), haemoglobin (RED) and carotene (YELLOW), which combine in varying amounts to make up your particular skin tone. You will either have a warm-based skin colour (Spring or Autumn) or a cool-based tone (Winter or Summer). If you have freckles they can help you find out if your skin tone is warm or cool-based: if the freckles are dark BROWN with a GREYISH charcoal appearance, your colouring is most likely to be cool; if they are GOLDEN YELLOW or light to medium BROWN with an ORANGEY look, your colouring is probably warm-based. Now look at the typical colouring of each season's skin, hair and eyes. Read the section you instinctively feel is right for you and check the details of your choice.

Winter

Skin   The predominant skin colouring of Winter is cool BLUE or BLUE-PINK. This may not always appear obvious immediately as it is often very subtle. Many people with Winter colouring have a GREYISH-BEIGE (TAUPE) skin-type ranging from light to dark, often with no visible colour (ROSE or PINK) in the cheeks. Some may be really quite sallow in complexion, and such people need the strong BLUE-based colours to counteract this.

There are more Winters than any other season, and thus more who need BLUE undertone colours to bring out the best in their natural colouring. Skin types include PINK as well; plain BEIGE or ROSE-BEIGE from light to dark; and OLIVE skins from light to dark – including cool-based BLACK- and BROWN-skinned people. Most people of African descent are Winter, although some may be Autumn.

Hair   Winter types often have dark hair, ranging from medium to dark BROWN or BLACK. Typical would be BLUE-BLACK or SILVERY-GREY or metallic ash, sometimes with a RED touch or highlight to it. Few Winter types are naturally blonde as adults, although many have blonde hair as children. If as adults their hair is blonde it is described as WHITE-blonde.

Eyes   The eyes of Winter types tend to show a strong contrast between the whites and iris colour. Winter eyes are often deep and clear. They may be BLACK-BROWN, RED-BROWN, BLUE or GREEN, GREY-BROWN or HAZEL. Sometimes HAZEL eyes with a lot of light-GOLDEN BROWN may seen warm in effect. Often Winter eyes have a GREY rim around the edge of the iris.

Summer

Skin   Summer people have a softer, more delicate colouring than that of Winter people. They often have a PINK colour in their skin which looks smooth, translucent and porcelain in effect. Many Scandinavians, Europeans and British people have a Summer complexion. They are fair and pale with a ROSE BEIGE or PALE-BEIGE skin, ranging from medium to deep.

Hair   Summer people often have blonde hair, ranging from WHITE blonde to GOLDEN blonde or ash blonde. However, when the Summer person ages, hair colouring tends to darken to ash BROWN with a GREYISH tinge. This is commonly described as 'mousey' colouring. Summer people with brunette hair may range from light to dark BROWN, also with GREYISH tones. Generally, Summer people's hair will go GREY gradually and softly, with a salt and pepper look.

Eyes   Summer types have eyes that are usually a misty BLUE, BLUE-GREY or soft HAZEL with BLUE-GREEN touches. They may also have soft warm BROWN or GREY BROWN in them, though the latter is not so common. The WHITES of the eyes are not sharp like those of Winter, but soft and CREAMY instead.

Spring

Skin   A Spring person has an IVORY, PEACHY PINK or GOLDEN BEIGE skin colouring. The skin has a ROSY glow to it, and often looks rather REDDISH. Freckles are typical of Spring people, usually with a GOLDEN colouring to them. But not all Spring types have freckles. Many have clear, CREAMY skin. The over-all warm colouring of Spring creates a bright and vibrant healthy appearance. Many Europeans, Americans and British people are Spring.

Hair Typical Spring people have blonde hair which often darkens with age. Flaxen blondes and GOLDEN blondes are all Spring, as well as many GOLDEN-dark-BROWN-haired people. Although not as common, it is possible to find dark BROWN/BLACK-haired Spring types as well. Some have an ash tone to their colouring, which can look drab. When the Spring person's hair turns GREY, it usually takes on a YELLOWISH tone. Dark BROWN/BLACK-haired Spring types turn SILVERY-WHITE, however, similar to that of Winter's GREY-haired people.

Eyes Most Spring eye colours are BLUE or GREEN or a combination of the two – (TEAL), TURQUOISE or AQUAMARINE, or BLUE-GREY. They range from light to dark. BROWN is the least common eye colouring for a Spring type; however, when it does happen, it is usually GOLDEN-tinged merging towards HAZEL, combining both GREEN and GOLD.

Autumn

Skin Autumn people often have a GOLDEN YELLOW undertone to their skin colour. There are three basic Autumn skin types: the fair person with IVORY to CREAMY PEACH skin; the RED-head with freckles of a GOLDEN TAN; and the GOLDEN-BEIGE-skinned person with tones ranging from medium to deep COPPER.

Many Autumn types lack colour in the face and tend to appear pallid or sallow. These people often look better in the dark, rich colours of the season.

Hair Autumn types can have hair ranging from AUBURN to COPPER, STRAWBERRY blonde to RED, dark GOLDEN blonde to warm BROWN, usually with a RED or GOLDEN highlight. Some, but not many, have CHARCOAL, BROWN or BLACK hair. In general, Autumn people do not go strikingly grey but in a more gentle way. Once their hair turns GREY it looks soft and warmly attractive.

Eyes Many Autumn people have dark BROWN or HAZEL eyes. Some have clear and bright GREEN eyes and are usually very striking, while others have deep OLIVE GREEN eyes with traces of BROWN in them. Just occasionally, Autumn types have bright BLUE or BLUE-GREEN (TURQUOISE) eyes but they do not generally have true BLUE or GREY eyes.

Personality, Colour and the Seasons

Through our work at Living Colour we have observed that there are distinct patterns connecting individual personalities with people's natural skin, hair and eye colouring and with the key colours in nature.

The relationship between these factors strongly influences the most appropriate colours to choose for clothes. For instance, take an individual who has a gentle, gracious personality, a ROSE-BEIGE complexion, ASH-BLOND hair and HAZEL eyes. There is a correspondence between the qualities of the personality (calm and gentle) and the colours (BLUE and PINK) of nature (Summer) (see Figs 10 and 11 on p. 102).

General guidelines for an understanding of the personality of each season are given below. They will help you to gain insight into the character of the seasons and show you how to relate to them personally.

The Winter Personality

Vivid contrasts and sharp colours are everywhere in the Winter months. Bare BLACK trees figure against the WHITE snow, creating a dramatic effect which is typical of the personality of Winter people. It is a quality which make them noticeable in a crowd; they are the kind of people who will be seen to have strong, self-assured manners in comparison with others. They can sometimes appear somewhat aloof, although many Winter people are actually deeply shy and often prefer the peace of their own company to being with others, limiting their circle to a few chosen friends.

They are good career people with big ambitions. They are reliable in a crisis, and despise disloyalty in others. They usually act fast once they have made a decision, and manage to get what they want in life, particularly in material terms.

Winter people are intelligent, good organisers, and make fine leaders.

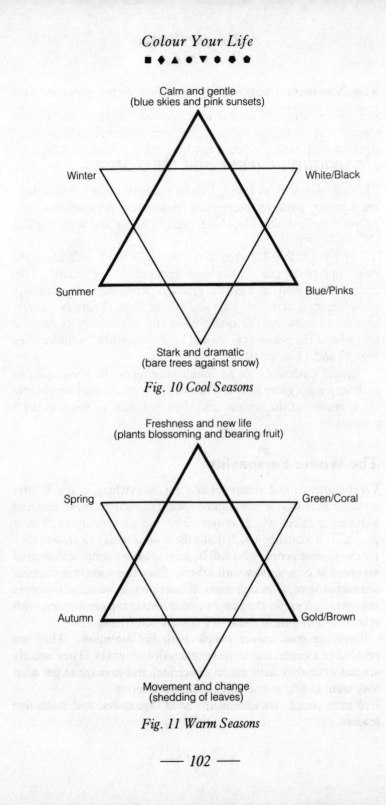

Fig. 10 Cool Seasons

Fig. 11 Warm Seasons

The Summer Personality

Summer people correspond with the soft, diffuse light of this season: they often appear as gentle, soft characters with a calm, gracious relationship to life. They have the constancy and dependability of the season, with its PINK sunsets and BLUE skies. The colours express comforting and reassuring qualities which are typical Summer traits.

Summer people are often perfectionists, who fail to achieve their high standards because they find it difficult to accept acknowledgement for anything they do. This leaves them without a sense of fulfilment and they try to compensate by being very analytical and criticising themselves and other people in roughly equal amounts. They are, however, good at listening to others, and they are always encouraging other people to improve themselves, while putting their own needs last. They will tend to deny themselves the opportunities they need to use their talents and in many cases they will withdraw and hide from life and miss out on the fun. These are frequently very serious people with a warm heart and deep feelings, but they find their feelings hard to express. They often lack spontaneity, and a basic willingness to participate in life.

Summers might be described as conservative, or reserved in character. They make very good, loving parents, and will be very well-organised domestically.

The Spring Personality

The basic colours of this season reflect the personality of people who are lively, vivacious and effervescent. Many of the colours in this season remind us of flowers and plants that bloom at this time and there is a warm, soft vitality about Spring people that is typical of this time of year.

Spring people are the opposite of the Summer type. These people are impulsive, easily responsive to the opportunities life offers, and they laugh a great deal. They are not, however, very well organised and often lack professional diplomacy. They will love to produce fresh ideas, but may typically have too many projects going at once, leaving them unable to deal effectively with any of them. However, Spring people will persevere in order to reach a goal. They make friends easily, and with their abundant natural good humour and energy, they get on well with most people.

Spring people are positive, optimistic and reflect the boundless, blossoming natural energies of the year's rebirth.

The Autumn Personality

With the changing of colours and the falling of leaves, Autumn signifies a return to the earth. Autumn types are earthy characters. These are independent, career-minded people who make good organisers and, unlike Spring people, can deal with many different projects at the same time. They are, however, quite temperamental, capable of both melancholic, depressive introversion and outgoing, fun-loving optimism. Autumn people like the company of others, but welcome solitude. They are an unpredictable group, but basically they are warm, friendly, loyal and lovable. They also make excellent leaders.

Types of Colour for Each Season

Each of the seasons contains four categories of colour: neutral colours, basic colours, bright colours and light colours.

Neutral Colours

The 'cool' Summer and Winter seasons have an undertone of BLUE/GREY of a varying intensity. In the 'warm' seasons of Spring and Autumn, the undertone is mainly BEIGE or BROWN, also varying in intensity.

The neutral colours are: WHITE, BEIGE, BROWN, GREY, BLACK and NAVY BLUE, depending on your season. These can be worn together with almost any other colour of that season. Neutral colours usually work to highlight or accent other colours in your clothes. They can also of course be worn as basic colours.

Basic Colours

Basic colours include certain kinds of RED, BLUE, GREEN and PINK in each season, ranging from medium to dark in tone. Basic colours have the effect of bringing colour to the face and are popular with most people whatever their season.

Bright Colours

Bright colours are the more intense tones of RED, BLUE, GREEN and PINK. As a rule, these strong, intense colours are worn best by those with a darker background colouring. Bright colours normally bring colour to the face, but if they are worn by those with a light background colouring then the effect can be draining. Bright colours work well for sports, on the beach and in accessories (handbags, scarves, belts and ties). They also work well in patterns such as floral designs and stripes.

Light Colours

These are the lighter tones of both the basic and the bright colours. They are the soft, delicate, pale colours which can be worn to good effect in blouses, shirts, underwear, scarves and handkerchiefs.

In this next section we will explain some of the basic qualities related to each of the seasons. We also include a table to help you create interesting colour combinations which could work for you.

WINTER COLOURS

Winter colours have a basic BLUE undertone. They are dramatic, vivid and sharp. ORANGE, PEACH, GOLD, BEIGE and BROWN together with YELLOW-based colours are best avoided altogether by those of this season. A Winter person should also avoid wearing muted or dusky shades, as these will subtract from their own natural colouring. The key colours for a Winter person are BLACK and PURE WHITE. For advice in combining colours, see below.

Winter Colours

Possible combinations

Neutral colours

Pure White	Blue, Red, Green, Grey, Pink
Black	Green, Turquoise, Red, Magenta
Grey	Red, Magenta, Green, Royal Blue
Navy	Red, Pink, Magenta, White, Grey
Taupe	Red, Maroon, Green, Black

Basic colours

True Red	White, Grey, Navy, Taupe, Black
Royal Blue	Red, Grey, White, Magenta
Magenta	Grey, White, Navy, Black Taupe, Green

Bright colours

Emerald Green	Grey, White, Black, Magenta, Pink
Clear Turquoise	Red, Magenta, Navy, White, Black, Blue
Royal Purple	White, Pink, Magenta, Lemon Yellow, White

Light colours

Lemon Yellow	Grey, Blue, Red, White, Black, Navy
Icy Pink	White, Black, Grey, Navy, Blue, Purple, Magenta
Lilac	Black, Grey, Navy, Blue, Purple, Magenta

Living Colour Wallets

The wallets supplied by Living Colour contain a wide range of different colours and other relevant information for each season. For more information see p. 182.

SUMMER COLOURS

All Summer colours have a GREY/BLUE undertone. Summer types
will look their best in soft, dusky, muted colours: this is basically a
romantic, charming effect whereas Winter is a very dramatic style.
Summer people will want to avoid BLACK or pure WHITE, which
will look harsh and rather stark on them. Instead, they can wear
cool BROWNS and soft CREAMY WHITES. The key colours for
Summer people are BLUES and PINKS. For advice on combining
colours, see below.

Summer Colours

Possible combinations

Neutral colours

Soft White	Cocoa Brown, Grey, Navy, Mid Blue, Rose Red, Pink, Plum Violet, Blue Green
Grey	Plum Violet, Navy, Mid Blue, Blue Green, Burgundy, Rose Pink, Sweet Pink
Rose Beige	Soft White, Cocoa Brown, Navy, Mid Blue, Lemon Yellow
Cocoa Brown	Soft White, Rose Beige, Silver Grey, Rose Pink, Fresh Yellow, Sweet Pink
Soft Navy	Grey, Soft White, Rose Beige, Mid Blue, Rose Pink, Yellow, Summer Pink

Basic colours

Rose Red	Grey, Soft White, Rose Beige, Yellow, Lavender, Summer Pink
Medium Blue	Soft White, Rose Beige, Cocoa Brown, Rose Red, Rose Pink
Rose Pink	Soft White, Navy, Grey, Blue Green, Aqua Turquoise

Bright colours

Blue Green	Grey, Rose Beige, Soft White, Lemon Yellow, Lavender, Summer Pink
Medium Blue	Soft White, Rose Beige, Cocoa Brown, Rose Red, Rose Pink
Sweet Pink	Soft White, Cocoa Brown, Soft Navy, Lavender

Light colours

Fresh Lemon Yellow	Navy, Cocoa Brown, Blue Green, Mid Blue, Rose Red, Soft White, Yellow
Lavender	Blue Green, Soft White, Grey, Navy, Plum Violet, Mid Blue, Rose Red
Summer Pink	Navy, Cocoa Brown, Mid Blue, Rose Red, Blue Green

SPRING COLOURS

Spring colours are clear, fresh, fruity and very vibrant. The predominating undertone is a warm YELLOW. Spring types should never wear BLACK, PURE WHITE, BLUE/RED tones, BLUE/GREEN or ROYAL BLUE which will all tend to substract colour from their faces, giving them a 'washed-out' look. Key colours for Spring people are CAMEL and CORAL. For advice on combining colours, see below.

Spring Colours

Possible combinations

Neutral colours

Ivory White	Milk Chocolate Brown, Camel, Navy, Lime Green, Turquoise, Red, Blue
Milk Chocolate Brown	Camel, Pink, Coral, Apricot, Peach, Turquoise, Lime Green
Grey	Navy, Violet, Red, Turquoise
Spring Navy	Camel, Grey, Ivory White, Pink, Red, Coral, Yellow, Navy, Apricot, Green
Camel	Ivory White, Brown, Red, Violet, Green, Turquoise, Blue

Basic colours

Spring Red	Ivory White, Grey, Red, Violet, Blue, Turquoise, Lime Green
Periwinkle Blue	Ivory White, Grey, Red, Coral, Apricot
Coral	Ivory White, Brown, Navy, Blue, Red, Turquoise

Bright colours

Lime Green	Ivory White, Grey, Camel Pink, Red, Violet, Golden Yellow
Spring Turquoise	Ivory White, Grey Red, Camel, Pink, Golden Yellow, Coral
Warm Violet	White, Grey Camel, Golden Yellow, Pink, Lime Green

Light colours

Golden Yellow	White, Grey, Navy, Camel, Red, Violet, Turquoise
Spring Pink	Navy, Brown, Spring Violet, Blue, Red, Spring Turquoise
Apricot Peach	Coral, Spring Red, Ivory White, Lime Green, Blue, Spring Turquoise

AUTUMN COLOURS

All Autumn colours have a YELLOW/GOLD undertone reflecting the autumnal colours of GOLD, ORANGE, YELLOW and EARTH BROWN. Autumn colours can be clear or somewhat muted. People who are Autumn types should normally avoid BLACK and the BLUE-toned colour range. Key colours for Autumn people are RUST and BROWN. For advice on combining colours, see below.

Autumn Colours

Possible combinations

Neutral colours

Oyster White	Brown, Cream Beige, Brick Red, Teal, Purple, Orange, Bronze, Mink, Olive Green, Rust
Plain Chocolate Brown	Oyster White, Cream Beige, Golden Orange, Yellow, Pink Salmon
Bronze	Cream Beige, White, Salmon Pink, Sun Yellow
Mink	Cream Beige, Oyster White, Teal, Orange, Green, Pink, Yellow
Cream Beige	Brown, Mink, Bronze, Olive Green, Rust, Teal

Basic colours

Rust	Cream Beige, Oyster White, Pink, Yellow, Sage, Olive Green, Teal
Olive Green	White, Beige, Bronze, Salmon Pink, Sun Yellow, Brick Red
Dark Periwinkle Blue	Oyster White, Cream Beige, Sun Yellow, Salmon Pink

Bright colours

Golden Orange	Teal, Red, Olive Green, Bronze, Mink, Brown, Beige, White
Autumn Teal	Salmon Pink, Oyster White, Brick Red, Rust
Autumn Purple	Pink, Sun Yellow, Sage Green, Oyster White, Cream Beige

Light colours

Sun Yellow	Brown, Mink, Bronze, Blue, Brick Red, Olive, Green, Teal, Purple
Salmon Pink	Brown, Mink, Bronze, Teal, Purple
Sage Green	Brown, Mink, Brick Red, Bronze

Clothes and the Colour Reflection

So far in this chapter, colour has been considered in relation to clothes and the personality of each season, from the point of view of aesthetics and the physical colouring of the individual. Wearing colour in clothes and being concerned about their decorative effect is both practical and pleasurable and it brings the energy of colour into continuous contact with our daily lives.

In terms of our health, however, the aesthetic use of colour is going to affect us on the external levels of our being only. In themselves, the colours of our clothes are unlikely to make a significant contribution towards the reduction of our physical ailments or our emotional imbalances. However, the use of colour counselling and colour therapy light treatment, which work on us internally as well as externally, are likely to increase our chances of establishing a balanced state of health. Even when you have discovered which season you belong to, and can choose the colours for your clothes in a systematic way, they will not necessarily be the colours which relate to your inner needs and the particular circumstances of your life at a given time.

To help achieve this level of relevance, you will want to combine the use of correct clothes colouring with your CRR and perhaps even colour therapy light treatment as well. Sometimes the colour/s you need for health at a particular time may not harmonise with your natural colouring. If this is the case you can work with the required colour through another medium. For example a Winter person requiring the colour ORANGE to help energise the physical body will find that this colour does not exist in their season. In this instance, the colour required can be worn as under-clothing or as accessories.

Introducing the colour/s you require in clothing is a positive step to bring more colour into your life, but of course it will only be a temporary measure, since we change our clothes every day. Added to this, the medium of colour in clothes is not potent enough to effect long-term benefical results. It can be a mild form of therapy which acts as a supplement to more advanced forms of colour therapy. It can help us to reaffirm or integrate particular patterns of energy which will influence our psychological and spiritual bodies.

Find out which season you are, and use this information as a

general guideline. Then, focus on the two colours you chose first
and second in your CRR. These represent your true self, and the
present conditions in your life. Wearing the colour of your first
choice is helpful to many people, since this colour will be in basic
harmony with your inner nature. Having understood the principle
of the CRR, you will then be in a position to apply colour in your
clothes, which relates to the second choice (or its complementary)
– i.e. your present circumstances.

Your third colour choice should be considered if it is in harmony
with either the first or second choice. In such cases, it should only
be used in small amounts, for accenting or highlighting the main
article of clothing. Here is an example of how this technique can be
used successfully.

Joanna – the case for violet
Our client Joanna was a health visitor by profession. She was tall,
slim, 29 years of age, with black hair, pale skin and HAZEL coloured
eyes. Joanna came to see us wearing a plain dark MAROON skirt, a
WHITE blouse and BLACK V-neck jumper. She was softly spoken,
articulate and wore black-rimmed glasses. The only piece of jewellery Joanna wore was an AMETHYST ring on her left middle finger.

She chose VIOLET as her first choice, MAGENTA as her second and
YELLOW as her third. Our advice, based on our interpretation and
the feedback we received, was that Joanna should wear the colour
VIOLET to help strengthen her personality, which appeared to be
weak. Since she did not wish to be colour analysed, she did not
know which season she belonged to. In this case the best we could
do was to recommend a colour, a deep VIOLET, that would suit her
natural colouring and with which we thought she would have a
natural affinity. Joanna felt unsure about this and so we suggested
that she could wear it in her underwear if she felt it to be too strong
near her face, or if she felt psychologically uncomfortable with it in
any way. She had never considered wearing VIOLET underwear,
and the idea held exciting possibilities!

We also decided that Joanna would need the colour of her second
choice, MAGENTA, and so we suggested that she used a deep shade
of MAGENTA where it merges with the deep VIOLET spectrum. The
combination of these two colours gives a beautiful colour called
FUSCHIA. We recommended that she wore this colour regularly for

a period of about three months. Since this colour was in itself quite close to the colour of her true self, it was one Joanna felt at home with. We then also suggested the use of YELLOW in her dress, since this was her third colour choice and is a colour harmony with her first choice. We suggested a deep VIOLET-coloured dress, with perhaps a soft YELLOW cardigan, or some form of accessory like a belt, scarf, necklace etc. It was important that Joanna wore predominantly VIOLET and only add small amounts of YELLOW, if she was going to introduce YELLOW at all. By doing this she would be introducing the colours of her true self with its complement which in Joanna's case would help to bring her goal closer.

Joanna rang us a week later to say that she had managed to find some VIOLET coloured underwear and a FUSCHIA coloured dress. She said, 'Initially I thought I wouldn't like them – but actually they look and feel very nice. I do feel positive and uplifted, and this seems to make me feel more confident about myself.'

When you know your season, the additional information offered by the Colour Reflection Reading will give new meaning to your colours. You will benefit by wearing the colours you need therapeutically as well as those that are physically suited to your natural colouring. If you are looking for something more than just 'what looks nice' in terms of colour, the CRR offers a wholistic and balanced approach.

Some companies and individual consultants involved in the colour-analysis business have approached us to help their students and consultants to understand more about the psychological aspects of colour and the therapeutic benefits which can be derived. Their interest developed as a result of their clients' strongly responding emotionally, either for or against the colours they were being asked to wear. Consultants trained in the therapeutic field of colour have much to gain in terms of the quality of service they can offer their clients.

It is important to make an accurate interpretation of the CRR, not only where there are emotional imbalances, but also where there are physical problems. The following example shows how the CRR was combined with a colour analysis for dress and colour therapy light treatment.

Judy – the need for blue

Judy was 28 years of age, trained as a graphic illustrator. She was about 5 ft 10 in tall, weighing approximately 9 st 8 lb and had a turned-up nose, big, HAZEL eyes, long eye-lashes and a long neck. Judy chose BLUE in the first position, RED in the second and TURQUOISE in the third.

Based on the interpretation and the feedback given by Judy, it became clear that for many years she had suffered from skin problems, in particular skin irritations, which often flared up, causing the skin to turn RED and blotchy. This was particularly so around the face, hands, feet and ankles. When we advised her to avoid the colours RED and ORANGE in her clothing Judy was disgruntled, since she was wearing a RED pullover. She said that she had a lot of RED clothes and thought the colour suited her, though she was indifferent to the colour ORANGE. Instead of RED, we advised her to wear BLUE and TURQUOISE clothes predominantly in order to help relieve the irritation and to calm and reduce the inflammation.

These were the colours of her first and third choices, but they also created the right therapeutic effect in her case. Judy felt comfortable and accepted our advice. Based on her physical health requirements and the CRR, we offered her colour therapy light treatment based on colour harmony – TURQUOISE harmonising with RED. TURQUOISE was administered as the therapy colour and RED as the complementary colour.

The next step of the consultation was to find out to which of the four seasons she belonged. Since she had BROWN/BLACK hair, HAZEL eyes and a medium-BEIGE skin tone, she was analysed as a Winter person. She needed the cool, BLUE-based colours to bring out the best in her natural colouring which also helped to reduce the RED patches on the face. When Judy saw for herself the effect of a RED drape against her skin, she could see how the existing RED blotches and patchy areas were heightened. She was amazed and fascinated to see how these areas were significantly reduced when cool BLUES, TURQUOISE and GREENS were put up against her. She was so intrigued by this that she asked us to repeat the process several times to check, as if she didn't believe it was true!

The suggestions and recommendations given to her were to keep away from the warm GOLD and YELLOW tone colours generally, as these colours would not uplift her natural colouring. She was also advised to avoid the cool tone REDS, MAGENTAS and PINKS within her season, as these are generally stimulating colours which would tend to inflame and irritate her condition. This is also true of ORANGE – though Judy didn't have to worry about this colour since it isn't included in the Winter palette. Even if the stimulating colours were basic BLUE undertone colours, the RED and PINK, for example, would still predominate and therefore would be unsuitable for Judy to wear.

From the CRR we know Judy has a true, BLUE personality (first position). We know that she suffers from skin irritation and inflammation which was her main physical concern at the time (i.e. negative RED in the second position), and was in need of its complementary colour TURQUOISE, which also happened to be her third choice. According to the colour analysis for dress, she is a cool-base Winter, with many of the personality traits that are also true for this season. She was now asked to prepare herself for the colour therapy light treatment. For this she needed to change into a neutral WHITE gown, and remove all synthetic fibres and any metal jewellery or other metal accessories. This she did and then sat in front of the Colour Therapy Crystal Light Unit, which projected the colours TURQUOISE then RED alternately, through a quartz crystal for approximately 20 minutes. (For more information on light treatments, see p. 87–9.)

About two months later (by which time her skin had cleared), Judy rang us to say how grateful she was for the whole consultation. It had made such a difference to her life.

chapter 6

INTERIOR COLOUR

The importance of interior colours and their influence on us becomes clear when you consider that on average we spend about two-thirds of our time indoors.

Colour is one of the major factors determining how we relate to our environment, and how it looks and feels. More than any other single element, colour can transform a drab, ordinary space into an enlivening one. Changing the colour of your walls can produce more dramatic results than changing the furniture or even altering the basic structure of the room. And, of course, it is far easier to do.

To make a personal colour connection with interior decoration, we must learn to overcome the fear of being different and unique, which often prevents people from 'playing' with colour and venturing out into a greater sense of self-discovery. Most of us have been conditioned to surround ourselves with 'sensible', 'quiet', neutral and pastel colours which inhibit our very existence and self-expression.

To help break through these inhibitions and make the most of colour in our environment, we need to discover more about our personal connections with colour and understand what the colours we like and dislike say about ourselves. By paying more attention to the power of colour in our homes, we may be pleasantly or unpleasantly surprised as to what it can reveal about us.

Simply consider the everyday things around the home. Start to become colour conscious by recognising the range of colours surrounding you. With this new awareness, go one stage further and look at the actual colours on the walls, ceiling and floor of the different rooms. How many times have you consciously stopped to question your reasons for choosing a particular colour scheme?

Look around the room you are in, and ask yourself what the colours say about you. You may feel there are too many colours surrounding you and somehow this creates a feeling that the room is closing in on you. Or that it appears too busy, demanding attention when all you want is to relax. On the other hand it could be that the room appears rather bland, colourless, without character, when what you'd really like is a room that reveals your adventurous and excitable nature. If you don't like what you see, you can consciously begin to alter the colours in your environment.

We could say that the colour of paint, wallpaper, fabric, carpet and other materials placed in a room are the garments covering the framework or structure of a building, just as the clothes worn by a person are the garments covering the skin, muscles and bones of the human body. Choosing the wrong colour in decoration can contribute to psychological and physiological imbalances. The effect of being exposed to it for long periods can be cumulative, making the problem worse. And since decoration is not something we change frequently, it is important to get it right, from the beginning.

There are two ways of looking at decoration: to be aware of the room in question and to focus on the colour you are using. Evidently, these two points of view overlap. Having separated them in your mind, remember to consider them both. Along with the preparatory process and the CRR they will lead you to your final colour choice. The following sections of this chapter work best when regarded as a whole, so try to use them as a springboard for your intuition and creativity and don't get too involved in the theory!

Preparing a Colour Scheme

The first thing to consider when choosing your colour scheme is your own personality. The information revealed through the colours you chose in the CRR (see Chapter 1) can now be used to construct a colour scheme specific to you. Other preparatory questions are as follows:

1. What kind of activity will be happening in this space?

2. How much light does it get? Is it basically a light or a dark area?

3. What kind of natural colour is there? Look at the wood, brick or stone.

4. Are you after a stimulating and bright environment or a calm and quiet one?

5. Do you want a basically cool or a basically warm atmosphere here?

6. Is there a high ceiling or a particularly low one?

7. Will you want to expand the size of this room or make it feel less large?

8. What is the basic shape of the room? Is it narrow and long or short and wide?

Suppose you wanted to decorate a room in colours that are strong, bright and stimulating. In general, these qualities tend to contract and reduce the apparent space of the room. RED, MAGENTA, ORANGE and YELLOW will give the effect you want, and these colours will work best in rooms where there will be a lot of activity. You might wish to decorate a kitchen, or part of the kitchen, in this way.

Other areas where strong, bright colour may be appropriate would be the children's playroom and the dining room. On the other hand, you may be looking for a softer, calmer and quieter environment. GREEN, TURQUOISE, VIOLET and BLUE will produce this effect. You might want to use these colours in your bedroom or a study area. They tend to promote feelings of expansiveness and openness.

Colour Terms

This section has been included to help you to understand the meaning of some everyday colour terms.

Primary Colours

Colour is a mental, emotional and physical experience. An account of what the eyes see and how the mind interprets this is both physiological and psychological and relates to each individual's spiritual and aesthetic connection with colour. This is far from the physicist's and chemical scientist's method of dealing with colour, as they are least concerned with the spiritual significance and more concerned with how colour involves compounds and pigments in both natural and artificial sources (from a chemist's point of view) and how the eye responds to colour involving light energy (from a physicist's point of view). In each area there are distinct laws as to the way colour will respond.

The *physics of colour* involves light and the primaries here tend towards white. There are three primaries: RED, BLUE/VIOLET and GREEN. The blending of RED and GREEN light, for example, gives YELLOW; GREEN and BLUE produce a clear TURQUOISE; and when BLUE and RED are combined they produce MAGENTA. The combining of the primaries in the physics of colour produces 'additive primaries' (see Fig. 12).

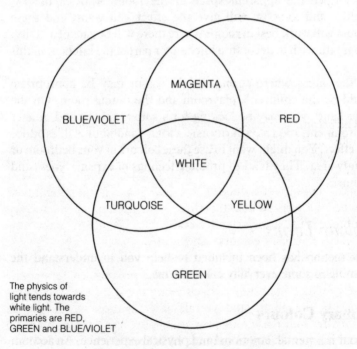

The physics of
light tends towards
white light. The
primaries are RED,
GREEN and BLUE/VIOLET

Fig. 12 Physics: Additive Colour Mixing

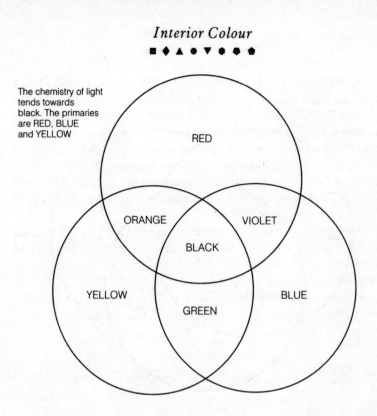

The chemistry of light tends towards black. The primaries are RED, BLUE and YELLOW

Fig. 13 Chemistry: Subtractive Colour Mixing

The *chemistry of colour* involves the use of pigments and compounds and involves three primary colours: RED, YELLOW and BLUE. When these are mixed together in varying combinations other shades occur, e.g. RED and YELLOW produce ORANGE; YELLOW and BLUE produce GREEN; and BLUE and RED combined produce VIOLET. When the three primaries of chemistry are combined they always tend towards black and are known as subtractive primary colours (see Fig. 13).

In the sensory aspect of colour it is a visual and mental concern. The human eye basically discerns four primary colours: RED, YELLOW, BLUE and GREEN. Each is unique and bears no resemblance to the others and yet all other colours are developed essentially from these four primaries, plus black and and white. Visual mixtures of these colours, excluding black and white, are medial and tend to work towards grey if combined (see Fig. 14).

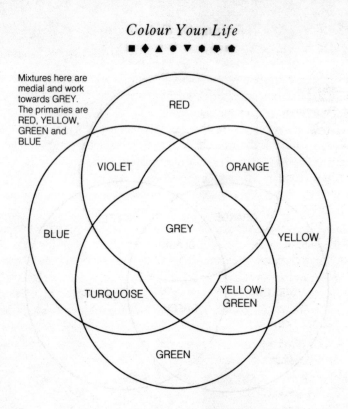

Mixtures here are medial and work towards GREY. The primaries are RED, YELLOW, GREEN and BLUE

RED

VIOLET   ORANGE

BLUE   GREY   YELLOW

TURQUOISE   YELLOW-GREEN

GREEN

Fig. 14 Primaries of Vision and Sensation

Depending on which medium you wish to work with, you would concentrate on the use of specific primaries of that medium. If you were to paint a beautiful picture you would use the laws of chemistry, applying the primaries of RED, YELLOW and BLUE. If you were involved in the engraving process of producing printing plates you would adopt the laws of physics and use the primaries of RED, BLUE and GREEN to bring about your desired affect. However, in the process of colour printing the primaries are MAGENTA, CYAN and YELLOW.

Hue

A hue is the attribute of a colour by which it is distinguished from another. It differentiates RED from BLUE, YELLOW from GREEN, ORANGE from MAGENTA. A hue also indicates a mixture of colours, such as ORANGE–RED (coral), YELLOW–GREEN (leaf green), or

BLUE–VIOLET (indigo). It can also be made from combinations of adjacent colours on the colour wheel such as RED/RED–ORANGE or BLUE/BLUE–VIOLET. All colours may be judged to be close to one, or a proportion of two, of the spectral hues, but they are distinguishable from each other. For example ORANGE, APRICOT and SALMON are close in hue, but are different colours.

Shades

Shadows and shades cause colour to change in appearance and tend to make them appear darker. For example a shaded RED is called MAROON, a shaded ORANGE is called BROWN, while a shaded YELLOW–GREEN is OLIVE. The effect of shading warm colours such as RED, ORANGE and YELLOW is profound in that the colour can change completely. For example RED darkened will appear almost BLACK; YELLOW darkened will change to GREEN, while cool colours such as GREEN, BLUE, VIOLET can appear to maintain their hues even with the strongest addition of shading. Therefore any colour mixed with BLACK will result in a shade.

Tints

The addition of WHITE causes the appearance of colours to change, tending to make them seem lightened. RED with the addition of WHITE is called PINK; ORANGE with WHITE is known as PEACH; and a lightened YELLOW–GREEN could be described as SAGE–GREEN or AVOCADO. Colours containing WHITE are known as tints. Colour terms such as powder and pastels generally refer to colours with the addition of WHITE. Colours which do not contain BLACK or GREY are tints and are often referred to as 'lively' colours because their intensity has been reduced with the addition of WHITE, causing them to appear lighter and more alive.

Tone

Intensity is not only dependent on the darkened or lightened quality of a colour, but also the degree of the tone. Tone can be described as a tint with BLACK present or a shade with a certain amount of WHITE. Another way of describing a tone is a colour where GREY is present, GREY being a colour created from BLACK and WHITE mixed.

Often colours containing GREY are termed 'tonal' colours, and are known as muted and dusky colours, or soft and dull. This is because these colours have an increased darkness or a reduced amount of WHITE which gives them this effect.

Colours which have been shaded are often referred to as 'deep' colours.

Lightening a shaded colour, or shading a lightened one, causes it to result in a GREYISH tone, while still maintaining a hint of the original colour (see Fig. 15).

Black

It is the basic nature of BLACK to absorb light. For this reason, it is the most effective way to contract space. It has a very dense, heavy

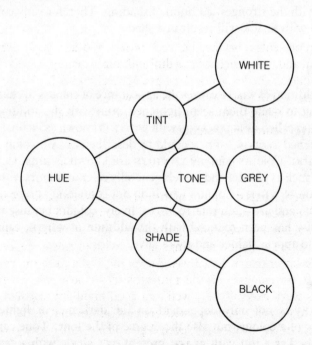

Fig. 15 The Colour Triangle

energy and it is not always easy to live with. For this reason, we suggest you use it in small amounts. BLACK is not recommended as a colour for ceilings and walls. One effective way of using it is to highlight woodwork, or furniture. BLACK mixes well with the pure hues and with any shade. But too much BLACK in decoration can produce a stagnant or negative environment.

White

WHITE is the opposite of BLACK in that it reflects light, and tends to expand space. If you are completely surrounded with WHITE, however, the atmosphere may feel rather cold and stark. WHITE can be used effectively as a colour for walls and for woodwork throughout the home. It will reflect hygiene, purity and cleanliness. A high percentage of people in Britain use WHITE around the house because of its ability to highlight and mix with other colours.

Grey

GREY represents a balance between WHITE and BLACK. It reflects caution, and is experienced as a dull and sombre energy. GREY, like all the darker shades, works best as a general highlight. However, medium to light tones work especially well on walls if accented by the use of bright colours for contrast or soft colours for a non-obtrusive, neutral environment.

Brown

BROWN represents the colour of the Earth and is related to stability. It reflects security, confidence and self-assuredness. The various warm tones of BROWN, ranging from very light to medium, tend to work well on walls, even ceilings, if you wish to create the feeling that it is lower than it actually is. Any of the LIGHT ORANGE, PEACH or APRICOT colours, or the LIGHT GREEN–TURQUOISE or TEAL colours work exceptionally well as a good highlight or balancing colour to BROWN. DARK BROWNS are best left to small areas in the home, as it can be too heavy, even depressing. DARK BROWNS work well out-doors, for example fencing, gates, garden sheds, walls, etc.

Ceilings, Walls and Floors

One very important point to remember when decorating is that colours generally seem to appear more intense in large areas than in small ones. Therefore we recommend, when covering a large area, to aim for a slightly lighter tint than the colour on the paint sample card.

It is good practice to make the ceiling a lighter colour than all the other colours in your room. This helps to conserve light, especially at night when there is no natural light source.

Traditional ceiling colours are WHITE or OFF-WHITE. However, if you want to lower a high ceiling, then you will want to choose a colour that is darker than the other colours in the room. Take care not to go too far. A lower ceiling can feel more intimate and homely, but too low an effect can be repressive and claustrophobic.

The traditional range of colours for walls goes from medium light to WHITE. The idea again is to make the most of available light, but if there should be an abundance of light entering a room, the darker shades will work instead. Extra artificial lighting in such a plan can dramatise and accent the space of the room.

Floor colours are normally medium to dark shades, or equal the lightness of the walls. The practical consideration tends to point to floor colours that are dark enough to absorb wear and tear, marks and stains. If you choose lighter floor colours, put them where the least traffic occurs, or where the least cleaning will be needed.

Rooms

The Living Room

Living room colours should be based on the existing natural colours. Floors, fireplace, brick or stonework should be considered as a starting point and any strong contrasts between dark and light shades should be avoided, because contrasts demand attention and the general purpose of this room centres on reading books, listening to music, talking and relaxing, from which you won't want distraction.

For interest we suggest you look for curtains or blinds which contrast slightly with the colour of the wall next to them. As a general principle, we suggest that sofas, rugs and chair coverings should be a darker shade than the wall colour. So, the basic plan for the living room involves a blending together of colour, without sharp oppositions. For effective highlights, think about the colour of the objects in the room, such as your vases, lamps and plants.

The Dining Room

Light to medium colours on the dining room wall will tend to create a happy, warm and welcoming space. We suggest that you look for these colours which relate to natural food colours. Where possible very pale colours such as pale GREENS and YELLOWS are best avoided as they can remind us of sickness and ill-health.

Contrasting colour can be used in small areas, such as the tablecloth, or the napkins. In general, look for the lighting levels which allow a clear vision of the colour presentation in the food.

The Kitchen

This room is rarely a place for relaxation. Plan your colours towards enhancing activity and focus on the warm end of the spectrum. These colours will support alertness, and stimulate creativity. Contrasting colours may be used on worktops, and this will help to raise light reflection in those places. Where darker shades are chosen, remember to provide strong, clear illumination. All your towels, china, saucepans and other kitchen equipment represent an opportunity to provide accents which relate to the principal colour of the room.

The Bedroom

This is a place for comfort and tranquillity. We suggest you choose soft, subtle colours rather than sharp contrasting ones, and heavy colours should be avoided. Think about the climate. In cooler countries, you will want to choose colours from the warm end of the spectrum. In warm climates, colours from the BLUE end of the range will be cool and refreshing.

Children's Rooms

For children up to the teenage years, we recommend colours from the RED, ORANGE and YELLOW end of the spectrum, to create a clear and bright environment. Above this age, the lighter tints of the GREEN and BLUE spectrums are often preferred. Dark colours should be avoided. Make sure to pay attention to lighting, so as to minimise eye-strain when reading.

Shared Bedrooms

When a bedroom is to be shared by a couple, see if you can find a colour scheme which is suited to both people. We suggest you avoid dark or vivid colours, unless you want to create a very strong or vibrant atmosphere, and focus on the soft, subtle tints such as ROSE, PEACH, soft LEMON, or LILAC and PINK which are warm and relaxing.

The Bathroom

Since bathrooms are usually small rooms, we recommend light to medium colours for the walls, in order to open up and expand the feeling of space. Tiles, sinks, baths and toilets are fairly permanent fixtures, and will probably be the starting point for the scheme. WHITE and OFF-WHITE shades are appropriate colours for the bathroom, since they tend to symbolise and encourage hygiene. Other suitable colours include any of the light to medium colours from the BLUE, TURQUOISE, BLUE–GREEN, AQUAMARINE or GREEN range. These symbolise the natural elements and reminds us of water, freshness and open space. Towels, toothbrushes, hairdryers, are all opportunities to add contrasting colour that relate to your general colour scheme.

Colour Qualities

As a general rule and a point worth remembering when using colour in decoration, as in any other media, is that over-exposure can create an imbalance just as under-exposure can. Colour must be used and kept in moderation to be sure of its constructive effects. The most harmonious results are achieved if you use the spectrum colours with their complementaries. Otherwise you could create the reverse effects to those initially intended.

Reds   This colour is appropriate for rooms where a lot of physical activity will be happening. Kitchens, playrooms, dining rooms, dance studios, discotheques and community halls can be highlighted with shades of RED with very beneficial results. RED is not usually appropriate where excitement needs to be avoided, as for example in a doctor's waiting room, a therapist's healing room or a study.

RED is the most dramatic colour in the spectrum, and should be used sparingly for the best effect. Be careful with the brighter hues of RED, which can produce an unsettled, tense effect. Dark shades of RED on the other hand can make the atmosphere seem unpleasantly heavy. Dark REDS are best used in small areas as a finishing touch. The pure hue of RED is rarely used as a wall colour, and should be especially avoided in workshop areas, or where there is a danger to people from tools and machinery.

Orange   This is made out of RED and YELLOW which gives it both the demanding qualities of RED and the lightness of YELLOW. It is more easily tolerated over large spaces than RED alone. It has an uplifting effect on the spirit, and provides a warm, soothing atmos-phere. Appropriate places to use orange shades would be kitchens, playrooms, living rooms and dining rooms, recreation rooms and hallways. Young children respond well to this colour, and wherever people get together to communicate or enjoy themselves, ORANGE is a wonderful colour to use. It promotes happiness and joy. Since the effect is similar to that of RED, it is not necessarily right for the study, the office or the bedroom, particularly in large amounts. There it can be used in its pure form on small areas of woodwork, such as window-frames, doors and skirting boards, or mixed with a little WHITE to create a pale PEACH or APRICOT tint.

Yellows   Excellent colours for the kitchen, especially when there is not much light available. YELLOW is a colour which pro-motes cheerful positiveness. The vibrant YELLOW range is not recommended for a study area. Associated with the intellect, it can have an overpowering effect on the mind over a long period, and promotes confusion. Intense YELLOWS are also not appropriate for bedrooms and living rooms, or any place which you intend as an area for relaxation. If you want to use the bright YELLOW shades in these places, we suggest that you try putting them with their complementary colour, which is VIOLET. VIOLET as the dominant shade will counteract any disorientating effect. If you go for the paler, more subtle tints and tones of YELLOW, such as BUTTERCUP, IVORY, MAGNOLIA or CREAM, the result will be less obtrusive. Paler YELLOW colours work well on walls. If you use the purer hues of YELLOW, then RED or ORANGE accents can be very interesting.

Green This is a serene, soothing colour which evokes natural surroundings. Light to medium GREENS, such as AVOCADO, LIME or SAGE GREEN can be very effective in the kitchen, except where there is little or no natural light. Darker shades of GREEN should normally be used sparingly as a general highlight on floors, cupboards or tiling. Areas which lead to the outdoors, like a courtyard or a conservatory work well in GREEN.

Since GREENS are basically calming colours they are often used to help neutralise tension. GREENS are helpful in hospital wards and operating theatres. In most stage theatres and opera houses there exists a GREEN room where the performers can relax and rest before and after the show. The darker shades of GREEN can have a draining effect if used over large areas. Anyone who finds it hard to get things moving in their life should avoid surrounding themselves with this colour.

Turquoise This colour produces feelings of coolness and freshness and aliveness. It is more versatile than GREEN. TURQUOISE expands the sense of space, and it works well in small rooms such as the bathroom or in waiting areas. Its BLUE content provides a peaceful, resting quality which evokes BLUE skies and seas. It is a direct contrast to our skin colour and works to enhance a glowing and healthy complexion. Used in bathrooms and bedrooms, it will reflect cleanliness and purity. TURQUOISE also works well in study areas and offices as a general colour for walls. The best wall colours for TURQUOISE are the light to medium tones. The whole range of

TURQUOISE from GREEN to BLUE can be used as an accent with most other wall colours.

Blues These colours lend themselves to calm, reducing stress, and so we always recommend them wherever rest, relaxation or peace is sought. BLUE can be used to great effect in rooms where prayer and meditation will take place. Lighter tints of BLUE work well in treatment rooms as well as in bedrooms, bathrooms and office areas.

As with TURQUOISE, BLUE is not very appropriate where physical activity is going to happen. In entertainment or dining areas it will present a cold and unfriendly ambiance, especially if the lighter shades are used. In general, light BLUES expand space and can be used to open up a confined room. As you move into darker shades of BLUE, the effect on your spirits can lead to laziness and melancholy, especially in large amounts.

Violet This colour promotes meditation and introspection. The lighter tints, such as LILAC, ORCHID or LAVENDER are very effective in treatment rooms, bedrooms or study areas. We recommend pale VIOLET for hospital waiting rooms, and recovery wards, where patients need to replenish their sense of self-respect and dignity. The VIOLET spectrum is associated with religious ritual and ceremonial occasions of all kinds.

Use VIOLET sparingly, especially when associated with the purer hues, where it will lead towards escapism and over-indulgence. Combined with the more intense, bright hues, the influence borders on oppression, especially at the psychic level. This combination is to be avoided where there is anyone suffering from instability or psychiatric disorders, where alcohol is consumed in large amounts, or where drug users congregate.

For safe results, consider carefully the relationship between VIOLET and the rest of your colour plan. VIOLET works well when complemented with the YELLOW spectrum.

Magenta This symbolises a nurturing, loving quality. The MAGENTA colours range from deep MULBERRY to a pale ALMOND blossom shade. They radiate warmth and affection, and work particularly well in an entrance hall and in bedrooms. MAGENTA is a reassuring protective colour to have around you. The lighter tints, which include ROSE, PINK and SALMON are popular bedroom and bathroom colours. PINK was found to be the most effective colour to apply on the walls of prison cells to help calm and soften inmates' difficult aggressive behaviour. However, when used as the predominant wall colours, they work well with the darker shades of MAGENTA, or with its complementary colour, which is GREEN. Examples of MAGENTA for highlighting include the darker tones and shades on woodwork, panelling, window and door frames, as well as in dining and living rooms.

MAGENTA in its pure hue is not usually very popular for offices, kitchens or study areas.

The Right Colours for You

In order to relate your choice of colour to your own specific needs, you must first refer to the Colour Reflection Reading. This is the key to an accurate assessment of those spectra of colours (i.e. the tints, tones and shades of your choice) that will work in harmony with your personality and needs.

Start with the three colours which you chose in the first chapter, referring especially to the first and third. We recommend you use one or a range of these colours, from the light (tints), medium (tones) and/or dark (shades), in those rooms you intend to decorate first.

Since the first colour chosen reflects your essential or true self, it will be in harmony with your basic nature. The third colour choice reflects the direction you need to move towards, and is recommended as the second most important colour you should consider. By applying these colours in your surroundings, positive qualities are more likely to be present in your home.

Should you be contemplating decorating more than two different areas, we suggest you choose a colour complementary to your first or third colour choices for the third area. The tints, shades and tones of these colours are most suitable. We do not usually prioritise the second choice since it reflects temporary situations and is subject to change. You can, however, use this colour range as an option, particularly in transient areas, such as halls, stairs and landings. All three colour choices represent the whole spectrum of each colour, ranging from light through medium to dark, so there is plenty of scope to experiment to achieve a beautiful environment that still relates well to your CRR.

Some Colour Schemes and How They Work

Claire is a 35-year-old actress with RED hair, BROWN eyes and a warm and cheerful disposition. She is about 5 ft 2 in tall with a petite frame and a lovely smile. She projected a pleasant personality, full of happiness. Her first choice was YELLOW, her second ORANGE and her third GREEN.

First choice (Yellow) Claire's 'bubbly' personality radiated warmth and light wherever she went, but although she was fun to be with, by the end of the session we found her personality quite tiring and mentally demanding. She seemed to be on a constant high. We felt she needed to learn to relax and slow down, especially on the mental level. We even wondered if her excessive verbal expression was in fact a nervous cover-up of a deep sadness of some kind or of depression. As it turned out we were right. Claire frequently experienced bouts of depression, and agreed that this depression might have been caused by her relying too much on her mental faculties and failing to follow her inner promptings. Claire tended to operate on an extreme vibration of YELLOW, which had the tendency to express itself negatively, constantly seeking logical and reasonable explanations to the situations in her life. She admitted that she frequently had good ideas, which she often seemed unable to apply in a practical way. This is a weakness typical of YELLOW people.

Second choice (Orange) This colour revealed a need to encourage more practical application of ideas. She needed to take a risk by venturing out of her mind and putting her ideas to work in a way that was truly grounded. She had a basic need for more confidence in her abilities. The colour also reflected the way in which she seemed to be depleted within herself, both mentally and physically. 'Being an actress is very demanding work,' she said.

We suggested that a challenge for her might be to take more time for herself, and replenish her energy overall. Only in this way could she develop the strength necessary to do what she always dreamed of in reality.

Third choice (Green)   This colour expressed Claire's need to find herself and work towards fitting in with the world. She said that she felt 'lost', and not being in a relationship and living on her own didn't appear to be helping matters. She felt insecure in her work because of its irregularity, and felt an especially important need to seek some emotional outlet. The energy of her third choice, GREEN, would supply some stability, and give her the space to make important decisions about her life. She had been seeing a counsellor to help her to explore her emotions in greater depth.

Advice and Suggestions
Claire wanted to know what colours would be best for her living room, bedroom and entrance hall. For her living room she brought along a sample of a fabric that was deep RUST-RED in colour. This was the covering of her sofa. She wanted to lay new carpet, and also paint the walls of the room, and asked us to help her plan a colour scheme for a room approximately 10 ft wide, 20 ft long and 10 ft high, with moderate light.

As she was naturally outgoing by nature, it was decided to go for the extrovert, warm end of the spectrum. Since her essential colour was YELLOW (the first card), these colours would have an uplifting effect that was in harmony with her true self. The question was: what kind of YELLOW would be the most appropriate for her needs? There is a big choice.

We advised her to choose a colour that would not produce too much stimulation or excitement – such as bold and vivid tones can do – but to choose one from the softer, more subtle tones which would have a gentle, warm and inviting effect. A light, unobtrusive tint would allow paintings, wall hangings and furniture to act as a highlight. She felt happy with this idea.

The next consideration was to decide on a colour for her floor carpet. We referred to the CRR again, using the third choice to give us an indication, taking her essence colour (YELLOW) into account. We advised her to go for a muted tone of deep SEA-GREEN, or BLUE-GREEN to balance the RUST-RED sofa and cushions and to

blend with the softly tinted YELLOW walls. We also suggested that
the carpet she might look for could be subtly mottled with varying
muted shades of GREEN and TURQUOISE. She was intrigued by this
combination of colours, and willing to follow our advice.

The next area Claire was looking at was her bedroom. This room
faced the garden, but received little sunlight. It was approximately
11 ft long, 8 ft wide and 10 ft high. Her bedroom already had a cool
medium BROWN coloured carpet, which was a base from which to
work. BROWN is a colour often associated with the earth. It is linked
with stability and groundedness and carries qualities of natural-
ness, durability and steadiness. Referring back to her essence
colour (YELLOW), and taking the preferred colour range for
bedrooms into account, we suggested she use a very soft LILAC or
pale LAVENDER for her walls. This would complement the brown
carpet, create a relaxing bedroom atmosphere, and act as a stabiliser for her personality.

So far, we had used the first and third of her colour choices for
her living room, and the complementary colour to the first colour
choice for the bedroom. This left the second choice to consider for
the entrance hall. The possibilities included the second choice
itself, its complementary colour, or the complementary colour to
the third choice. This brought us to a choice between tints of
ORANGE, BLUE, or MAGENTA. MAGENTA was not a colour she felt
drawn to, while BLUE was not recommended because of her tendency to depression. The complementary to her second (ORANGE)
colour choice was BLUE, which could promote a melancholic
atmosphere, which we wanted to avoid. Finally we recommended
a colour from the ORANGE spectrum we felt would be just right. A
soft tint of PEACH–APRICOT.

Claire passed by our stand at an exhibition about a year after she
came for her Colour Reflection Reading. She expressed how she
had applied the colour advice we gave her and found the YELLOW in
the living room very pleasing. She said that she particularly liked
the light and happy atmosphere the YELLOW walls seemed to
create. The carpet she finally managed to get contained a mixture
of softly muted BLUE, GREEN, PINK and VIOLET, which she felt
worked very well. 'I am increasingly coming to terms with the
LILAC colour in my bedroom. One thing is for sure, I do seem to be
sleeping better! In the hall the soft PEACH–APRICOT colour always

gives me a lovely welcoming feeling when I get home, especially in the winter. I'm very happy with the outcome.'

Now it is your turn to experiment. Don't be afraid to be creative, and use your imagination!

chapter 7

■ ◆ ▲ ● ▼ ● ◆ ◆

COLOUR IN
BREATHING,
VISUALISATION AND
AFFIRMATION

In this chapter, we will look at some powerful techniques which use colour to explore our inner selves and influence both the creative imagination and the unconscious mind. Breathing, visualisation and affirmations are excellent stress-relieving methods and can be practised together as the Creative Colour Technique, or used independently. We suggest you get familiar with each one, approaching them separately to begin with.

First you need to develop the technique of deep breathing. This can take a little practice, and though at first you may feel quite awkward, it will soon feel entirely natural. We will then describe how to extend this to colour breathing. The exercise can be made specific and personal to you by integrating the positive qualities of your second colour choice from your Colour Reflection Reading.

The colour visualisation process allows you to focus on a particular aspect of your life that you might not be happy about, beginning by isolating exactly what it is you feel unhappy with. By having acknowledged that something is not quite right, you have already started to remedy it.

The steps towards attaining your goal are fully explained, and as you focus on this and see your goal materialise, you will also in effect be working with the colour of your third choice. For example, a person who feels 'unlovable' might visualise being surrounded with special friends who are showing them love and affection. To do this you will work with the energy of the colour MAGENTA, and to further the process you could imagine the whole scene taking place in a sphere of MAGENTA light.

The third part of the chapter is devoted to colour affirmations. These are positive, affirmative statements which are repeated regularly in order to produce a specific result. They derive from your own specific needs, as revealed through the CRR. This process uses colour in the environment as a trigger to help remind you of what you wish to attract and create in your life. Since colour is everywhere and all around us, this also becomes an enjoyable way to develop your awareness of colour and appreciate its richness.

The final section of this chapter explains the stages involved in bringing all three elements together into the integrated Creative Colour Technique.

Breathing

Breath is life. From the cutting of the umbilical cord, breathing is so vital to us that we cannot survive without it for longer than a few minutes. And with the breath of life comes the energy which stabilises, sustains and revitalises our body. Hindus call this energy Prana, and the Prana, or life force, which is available through breathing deeply and rhythmically is not confined to the lungs. Our breath is drawn from deep within the belly, as well as through the pores of our skin. Where there is perspiration, there is also inspiration! With the help of a little visualising you will be able to relate more fully to this kind of breathing.

In order to breathe properly we need to be free from tension and completely relaxed. Few people have a deep rhythmical and relaxed breathing pattern. Instead breathing tends to be shallow, with a tendency to hold on to the breath. This usually produces a succession of short, quick, inefficient breaths which in time can cause the lungs to atrophy. In order to keep the lungs working and the diaphragm functioning healthily, it is important to include deep breathing as part of any colour breathing and colour visual-isation exercise.

Pause now for a few minutes, and you can experience this for yourself. First, sit comfortably and let your whole body gradually relax, focusing on your breath. Allow yourself to become aware of the inhalation and exhalation, without attempting to force the breath in any way. Just allow it to take its own course and speed. And as you begin to relax, consciously imagine the breath passing though every pore of your skin as you breathe, simultaneous with the respiration, in and out. Notice how this visualisation feels to you, and how your body responds to it. You can practise this form of breathing whenever you feel like it. Now put the book aside and try it for a few minutes with your eyes closed.

This exercise has the effect of improving our breathing pattern so that we are able to absorb the precious Pranic energy more fully. Perhaps we have neglected to pay attention to the way we breathe because breathing is a partly involuntary process and happens automatically. Bad habits such as sitting in a slumped posture, rushing around and smoking will contribute toward basically unhealthy breathing patterns. Over long periods, the cumulative effect produces irregular, weak and shallow breathing which can be physically draining, and lowers our resistance to infection and sickness.

A Simple Breathing Exercise

This simple breathing technique, if practised regularly, will help you to breathe deeply and rhythmically, and will contribute to your overall health and vitality. When learning to breathe properly it is important not to try to 'force' the breath in any way. In other words, do not try to lengthen your breathing artificially, or 'hold' your breath. This is especially relevant if your breathing is shallow or weak to begin with. Allow the breath to move naturally, smoothly and gently. With practice, it will gradually strengthen, deepen, and lengthen as well.

To begin with, focus on releasing as much air as you comfortably can with each out-breath. This will contribute towards the process of cleansing the body, by eliminating residual or stagnant toxic substances. As you make progress with the breathing, allow the out-breath to last a little bit longer than the in-breath. This is a much more effective way to breathe than taking short quick breaths.

By breathing deeply and consciously in this way you awaken and stimulate the solar plexus region, which is connected to the central nervous system. This centre is also referred to as your 'power' centre. Once you have made contact with it through your breath, you will be able to feel the power of your body more and more easily.

Here is the procedure for deep, rhythmic breathing. Read it through before practising the exercise.

1. Become conscious of your breathing.

2. Breathe in from the solar plexus by extending the belly outwards while you inhale. Then draw the breath up to the chest.

3. As the breath rises, expand your chest sideways instead of forward as you normally do.

4. When you have inhaled as far as you comfortably can, holding the belly out, allow a moment's pause.

5. During the exhalation that follows, pull your belly in and then relax the chest, remembering to release as much air as possible.

6. Repeat these steps five times.

Be aware of keeping your shoulders relaxed throughout the exercise. For the best results, we recommend you practise in a clean, fresh environment such as out of doors, or near a window, first thing in the morning.

Colour Breathing

Colour breathing is a way of relating the energy of colour with the rhythm of the breath. By doing this we can literally charge the breath with colour energy, making it more potent and directing it for specific purposes. Apart from the innate benefits of breathing deeply, the use of colour can channel and direct Prana for harmony and healing. This is accomplished through the chakra system, and by breathing while visualising specific colours you will also improve the general state of the chakras themselves.

In order to use colour breathing effectively, it is essential that you become adept with the deep breathing exercise. This means you must be able to breathe naturally in the way we have described, without thinking out the movements. Once you have accomplished this, you can start to use colour as well. One of the main benefits of colour breathing, apart from its relaxing and revitalising effect, is that you will become more aware of physical and emotional imbalances and be able to influence them positively. In this way we can consciously effect change and healing where there is negativity or dis-ease.

The colour breathing exercise

It helps to have your eyes closed when practising this exercise, in order to focus inwardly and avoid distraction.

1. Find a comfortable position and sit or lie with the spine straight and the soles of the feet on the ground, slightly turned inwards.

2. Close your eyes and begin to breathe deeply and rhythmically. Imagine a shaft of pure WHITE light entering through your head from the cosmos down to the extremities, engulfing your entire body inside and out, and then leaving through the soles of your feet.

3. Now try to imagine a sphere of PINK MAGENTA light surrounding the top of your head (the crown chakra). Breathe in this nurturing, warm colour five times.

4. Move your attention to the centre of your forehead slightly above the eyes (the third-eye chakra) and breathe in the healing colour VIOLET. Repeat five times.

5. Move on to the area of the throat chakra, and breathe in the serene colour BLUE. See it emanating from the centre of the throat as you exhale. Repeat this five times.

6. Allow your attention to move to an area mid-way between your heart and your throat (the thymus chakra) and breathe in the refreshing, sparkling colour TURQUOISE, five times.

7. Now move to your chest (heart chakra) and feel it expand with the soothing colour of GREEN. Repeat five times.

8. Imagine a GOLDEN YELLOW light around your middle (the solar plexus chakra) and breathe in this gloriously radiant colour deeply. Repeat this five times.

9. Next, bring your attention to the lower abdominal area (the spleen chakra) and breathe in the joyous, vibrant colour ORANGE, five times.

10. Now move to your pelvic area (the base chakra) and imagine the vital colour of RED around this region. Breathe in this colour five times. The energy from the pelvic area downwards should be imagined as WHITE light flowing down through both legs and gathered at the soles of the feet. Allow this energy to seep into the ground like the roots of a tree, earthing you and stabilising you as it does so.

11. Finally imagine breathing in pure WHITE light which surrounds you from head to toe in every direction and flooding your entire organism, inside and out.

Throughout this exercise, see the colours become clearer and more vibrant with each breath. This is a wonderful exercise for relaxation which can be practised anywhere, whenever you have the time, even on the bus, or on the train home. To make the colour breathing exercise more immediately relevant to your present needs, simply introduce the positive attributes related to the colour of your second choice in the Colour Reflection Reading. Using the deep breathing method, you start to see the colour of the second choice with each in-breath and with each out-breath exhale the dark and murky aspects of this colour.

Should you have difficulty seeing the colours throughout the colour breathing exercise, simply recall an item or an object that reminds you of the colour you are trying to see. For example, if you had difficulty seeing a sphere of PINK MAGENTA light, perhaps the image of a favourite PINK jumper or a summer rose will help you to make the association.

When colour breathing is put together with colour visualisation and colour affirmation, which are described later in this chapter, you should use the colour of your third choice in place of the second as you now need to relate to your *future* needs.

Colour Visualisation

Visualising is a way of using the imagination to create pictures in the mind with the intention of attracting what we want into our lives. In fact this technique is something we use constantly, although we are not usually aware of it. Most of the time we use mental images to create and reaffirm whatever deep-seated beliefs we already hold about life. Some of these are necessarily negative and limiting to us (as they assist us in our growth), and express themselves in the form of failings, difficulties and even ill-health. It is clear that if we constantly imagine problems and project our negative beliefs into our lives, they will tend to become a reality. And, to use an analogy, if we plant corn, there is no way we are going to reap turnips.

Colour visualisation is about acknowledging the negative thought patterns which already exist, and starting to replace them with new and positive ones supported by the energy of colour. It is a process of planting positive images, in order to reap positive results. It is necessary to approach the whole process with both an open mind and a willingness to try it out and see what happens. It is not necessary to believe in any spiritual force or external powers, but only to focus on your own personal power to achieve your desired goals. In order to define these goals more clearly, it will help you to make a detailed written statement of what you want. It is important not to be vague.

Let us say, for example, that you are unemployed and having difficulty finding a satisfactory job. You should therefore decide what kind of job you would like to have, how much money you want to earn, and to consider holidays, travelling (distance and time), as well as the exact responsibilities and duties you will be taking on. Here the predominant colour energy is TURQUOISE, the colour of change and of clarification.

As with any new concept, a good place to start is with a fairly easy task. Choose one that you feel is well within your capabilities; accomplishing this goal will add to your confidence and make it possible for you to attempt more difficult ones later on. Once you have defined this goal in detail, the next step is to create a clear picture of it in your mind. For this, you will need a quiet place, and for the best results we advise you to practise with your eyes closed. You need to visualise whatever it is you desire or want in detail, and see yourself already in possession of it. Bring all your senses into play to make your goal as realistic as possible to you, in any way that comes naturally.

An example, if you wanted to improve your social life by making more friends, you might practise seeing yourself in the company of others, and enjoying yourself with them. You could also imagine how others enjoy your company. If you are the sort of person who tends to observe others and hold back in company, try seeing yourself initiating conversations instead. Eventually this will become a reality in your life, provided that you practise the exercise frequently, with the conviction that you really deserve your goal. The colour energy here is ORANGE, which reflects the above.

Next, ask yourself what you are prepared to give in order to achieve your objective. This giving might take the form of discipline, persistence, or dedication. Ask yourself: 'How much am I willing to give in order to achieve my goal? What kind of effort am I ready to make?' Having decided what you are prepared to give to achieve your goal, you must start bringing the image of what you desire frequently to mind. This is a form of acknowledgement which will assist you. Beware, however, of yearning and longing and wanting your goal 'too much'. Over-emphasis will only tend to push it away instead. Your desires must be approached in a gentle and relaxed state of willingness. This is an attitude which works. As your goal becomes an increasing part of your awareness, direct positive and encouraging thoughts and energy towards it. Affirm to yourself that your goal is increasingly becoming a reality for you, that it exists in your future, that it is out there waiting for you. It is very important to acknowledge any doubts or hesitation that you may have in relation to your object, since these will obstruct you from achieving what you wish if remained unexpressed.

In order to link your visualisation with colour energy, allow yourself to bring in the qualities of the third colour that you chose in your CRR in to your natural surroundings while you visualise your goal. For example, a client came to us who had a marked tendency to withhold his feelings. As a result of this, he also tended to feel 'trapped' inside himself. We suggested that he used visualisation to start seeing himself as a person who is able to express emotions freely. This in fact accurately reflected the quality of his third choice (GREEN), and the general goal in his life at this time.

Summary of the Colour Visualisation Process

1. Start with a simple goal in order to familiarise yourself with the process. Achieving this will add to your confidence.

2. Define exactly what it is you want to achieve and concretise it by writing down a detailed description. Doing this makes the goal specific and contributes towards materialising it.

3. With your eyes closed create a clear picture of your goal. Imagine yourself already in possession of it. Use your senses to make it real to you.

4. Decide what you intend to give in order to achieve your goal.

5. Focus often on your goal, to strengthen your purpose.

6. Continue to practise until you have either achieved your desire, or until you no longer wish to achieve it. You, or your goal, may change!

Points to Remember

1. Be consciously aware that what you choose is what you really want to realise.

2. Be prepared to change directions and be flexible. Stay with what is happening in every moment. You may need to take detours, before reaching your goal.

3. Commitment and perseverance are essential for a successful outcome.

4. Monitor your goal to make sure it is still what you want.

5. When you feel, think, or experience anything negative, translate it into something positive.

6. You can only learn from your experience and so there is no way you can fail, even though this may not be apparent at all times!

7. Reward yourself for your successes in a clear and noticeable way. Give yourself a pat on the back by treating yourself to some special pleasure.

8. Enjoy the whole experience, and make it fun.

First Aid Guide

Here is Living Colour's first aid guide to healing through colour visualisations. Use this technique alongside orthodox treatment to speed up your recovery.

Ailment	Colour	Ailment	Colour
Abcess	Turquoise	Cold	Red/Orange
Acne	Turquoise	Cold sore	Turquoise/Blue
Agoraphobia	Orange/Red	Conjunctivitis	Blue/Violet
Alcoholism	Orange	Constipation	Orange/Yellow
Anaemia	Red	Cough	Blue
Angina	Green	Cramp	Blue
Anorexia	Orange/Blue	Cyst	Green/Magenta
Anxiety	Blue	Cystitis	Magenta
Arthritis	Yellow/Orange		
Asthma	Turquoise/Blue	Depression	Orange
		Dermatitis	Turquoise/Blue
		Diabetes Mellitus	Yellow
Backache	Blue	Diverticulitis	Orange
Bladder problems	Orange	Dyspepsia	Orange
Blisters	Blue		
Blood pressure		Earache	Blue/Violet
– high	Blue/Turquoise	Eczema	Turquoise
– low	Orange/Red	Emphysema	Green/Blue
Boils	Turquoise	Epilepsy	Blue/Violet
Bronchitis	Green/Blue		
Bruises	Blue	Fatigue – mental	Turquoise
Burns	Blue	– emotional	Green
		– physical	Blue/Orange
Cancer	Green/Magenta	Fainting	Magenta/Pink
Cataract	Green/Blue	Fever	Turquoise/Blue
Catarrh	Turquoise/Blue	Flatulence	Blue
Chest pain	Green	Food poisoning	Yellow/Turquoise
Claustrophobia	Green	Frostbite	Orange/Red

Ailment	Colour	Ailment	Colour
Gallstones	Orange/Blue	Muscular dystrophy	Yellow
Gastric ulcer	Green	Myopia	Blue/Violet
Gastroenteritis	Turquoise	Multiple sclerosis	Yellow
German measles	Blue		
Glandular fever	Blue		
Gout	Orange/Blue	Nausea	Magenta/Blue
		Neuralgia	Blue/Violet
Hay fever	Turquoise/Blue	Nosebleed	Blue/Violet
Headache	Blue/Magenta	Numbness	Red
Heartburn	Green/Magenta		
Heart disease	Green	Oedema	Blue
Heart-palpitations	Green/Magenta	Ovarian cysts	Magenta/Green
Haemorrhoids	Turquoise/Blue	Paralysis	Red
Hepatitis	Yellow	Paranoia	Violet
Hernia	Blue	Peptic ulcer	Green
Herpes simplex	Blue	Peritonitis	Blue
Herpes zoster	Turquoise/Blue	Phlebitis	Blue
Hiccups	Blue	Pleurisy	Green/Blue
		Pneumonia	Turquoise/Blue
Indigestion	Blue	Pre-menstrual syndrome	Blue
Inflammation	Turquoise/Blue		
Influenza	Blue		
Itching	Blue	Raynaud's disease	Red/Orange
Insomnia	Blue		
		Respiratory problems	Blue/Orange
Jaundice	Yellow		
		Rheumatism	Yellow/Orange
Kidney disease	Orange		
		Scarring	Blue
Laryngitis	Blue	Schizophrenia	Yellow/White
Leukaemia	Red	Sciatica	Blue/Violet
Liver disease	Yellow/Orange	Shock	Magenta/Green
Lumbago	Blue	Sinusitis	Turquoise/Blue
Lung problems	Green/Blue	Skin problems	Turquoise
		Sneezing	Blue
Measles	Blue	Sores	Blue
Menopause	Violet/Magenta	Sprains	Blue
Mental illness	Violet	Stammering	Blue
Migraine	Magenta/Blue	Stiffness	Orange/Yellow
Morning sickness	Magenta	Stings	Turquoise/Blue
Mumps	Blue	Stress	Turquoise/Blue

Ailment	Colour	Ailment	Colour
Stroke	Magenta	*Ulcer*	
Sty	Blue/Violet	– *of stomach*	Orange
Sunburn/	Blue	– *of duodenum*	Blue
Sunstroke		*Urinary*	Blue/Orange
Swellings	Turquoise/Blue	*infections*	
Toothache	Blue	*Varicose veins*	Blue/Violet
Tension	Turquoise/Blue	*Vertigo*	Magenta
Thrombosis	Blue	*Vocal problems*	Blue
Thrush	Blue	*Vomiting*	Magenta/Green
Thyroid			
– *overactive*	Blue	*Warts*	Green/Violet
– *underactive*	Orange	*Wheezing*	Blue
Tinnitus	Blue/Violet	*Whooping Cough*	Blue
Tiredness	Blue/Magenta		
Tonsilitis	Blue		
Trauma	Green/Magenta		
Travel sickness	Blue		
Tuberculosis	Green/Turquoise		
Tumours	Green/Magenta		

Colour Meditations

Colour visualisation exercises can be used as a form of meditation in order to create positive, healing and uplifting effects, or purely for pleasure. Since meditation brings good health and balance to the physical, emotional and mental bodies, the aura itself is revitalised by the act of meditating. The following meditations for each colour are based on the colours found in nature. It doesn't matter if in real life you haven't actually seen or experienced the sights described in the following meditations. What is more important, is how far you allow yourself to go with your imagination to picture the scene, as if it were actually happening. Try as much as possible to make the image of the scenes described as lifelike as possible, as if you were experiencing it for the first time.

Colour in Breathing, Visualisation and Affirmation
■ ◆ ▲ ● ▼ ● ● ●

The following colour meditations are like a journey. Each one should last for approximately 20 minutes and can be used any time during the day. Use them for pleasure and to help you to heighten your awareness of each colour and their associated qualities. They can also be used according to your personal needs and to counteract a specific mood. For instance, if you are 'feeling BLUE', try the ORANGE SUNSET mediation, or even the YELLOW SUNFLOWER meditation to help uplift you. If on the other hand you are feeling stressed or hyperactive, the BLUE SEAS meditation would probably be your best choice. (See chart – The Living Colour Guide to Colour and Its Effects on page 148.)

One point worth mentioning here regarding meditation practice is that many people (especially those new to meditation), tend to be put off by an inability to concentrate. Throughout your meditation take regular moments to pause in order to absorb your experiences fully. Deep rhythmic breathing is very useful to help keep you centred and 'on track'.

If for any reason unassociated thoughts or images not linked to your meditation should come into your mind, very gently try to put them aside and continue from where you left off. The experience of so-called 'interfering' thoughts and 'distractions' are common and you should try to avoid them where possible. They should not be encouraged during meditation practice as this will only take you further away from your meditation and lead you to be mentally active. But such experiences are not necessarily negative: they can be seen as a subtle way the body releases stress and tension, normally held buried within the system. So if this happens to you, relax, let go of the distractive thoughts and/or images, and return naturally to your point of focus and continue your meditation. The ability to focus and concentrate without distractions comes with regular meditation practice, which will help to keep you free from stress.

Now read through the eight colour meditations, choose one according to your present needs, and practise colour meditating. You may find it helps to record your meditation slowly on to a tape in your own way and play it back to yourself. This will enable you to relax and experience it more deeply.

The Living Colour Guide to Colour and its Effects

Colour	Chakra	Psychological effects	Physiological effects
RED	Sacrum	Stimulates and increases alertness	Raises blood pressure and releases adrenalin
ORANGE	Adrenals	Cheerful encourages joy	Aids digestion and metabolic system
YELLOW	Solar plexus	Positive and bright	Nervous disorders
GREEN	Heart	Harmonious and balancing	Heart and chest conditions
TURQUOISE	Thymus	Refreshing and cool	Relieves pain and is anti-inflammatory
BLUE	Thyroid	Peaceful and calming	Reduces blood pressure and relieves throat problems
VIOLET	Pituitary	Encourages inner awareness	Purifies body and aids sleep
MAGENTA	Pineal	Love and compassion wholeness	Relieves migrane and headaches

Red Fire

It is a cold Winter's evening and you are comfortably reclined in your favourite armchair which is positioned slightly to the right of a burning log fire. The lights are dimmed and the room is aglow. Your attention is focused on the fireplace in front of you. The flames flicker and dance in different shades of RED, creating shadows against the RED brick background. As the strength of the fire burns, the glow of vibrant light shines out and radiates on your face. You are warmed and comforted by the heat generated from the crackling, burning wood. You gently nestle your tired body deep into the soft cushions supporting your back and absorb the penetrating heat through every part of your body.

The flames seem to speak to you, luring you to come closer. You respond by focusing deep into the heart of the fire, gazing and admiring the power and strength that it offers. You take a deep breath and begin to feel energised and awakened. You marvel at the spectrum of flame colours; deep RED, CRIMSON, SCARLET and sizzling VERMILLION. The intensity is almost too much to bear; your heart begins to throb, excited by the increasing power and light that permeates the very core of your being. Charged with an incredible force, and will to live life to the full, you realise your potential to radiate warmth, love and friendship with all those with whom you come into contact.

Orange Sunset

You are sitting in a chair, on the veranda of a house on the top of a cliff, overlooking the sea. It is late August – about 7.30 in the evening – and the sun is soon to set. As you look out to sea, you reflect on the events of today. You recall the joy of reuniting with friends you hadn't seen for a long time and how much fun and laughter you shared together. You remember their smiling faces and the happiness in coming together. In your hand is a cool, refreshing drink: you take a sip and once again look out into the distance.

The sun is about to set beyond the horizon. A giant ORANGE disc in the sky moves slowly, sinking inch by inch to kiss the sea. Like a hole in the sky, it burns, radiating its light upon the waves of the ocean, caressing the water and glittering like sequins on an evening dress. The sky is aflame with GOLD, APRICOT and ORANGE streaks, interspersed with soft shades of complementary colours. Your eyes light up and sparkle in the radiant glow of the sun's rays. As it passes halfway beyond the horizon, its reflection seems to turn the sea to fire, rejoicing at the splendour of life and the vitality it gives.

You think back to your friends, remembering how as each of you parted, you promised to keep in touch and meet more often. The busy sounds of people talking and children playing and splashing in the sea have now ceased. There is expectancy in the air. For a brief moment there is silence all around. If a pin dropped now, you would hear it hit the earth. The GOLDEN ORANGE globe is about to slip away and disappear beyond the horizon and out of sight. The last shimmering view of this exuberant ball in the sky melts in the distance. Only the memory of the evening fire is left with you now. At least until tomorrow.

Yellow Sunflower

Picture yourself walking through a field of sunflowers, most of which have grown to the height of approximately six feet. The stems are GREEN, thick and rough; the leaves are coarse and grow from offshoots interspersed along the stem. The heads are big and round with bright GOLDEN YELLOW petals, embracing the complex centres, which are a network of honeycombed sockets filled with seeds and covered with a thick MUSTARD-YELLOW layer of fine hairs, tipped with pollen. Each petal is soft and velvety to touch. They are long and thin and slightly rounded at the tip. You gaze into the centre face of one of the sunflowers and realise the amazing structure and ordered pattern contained within. You are awed by its beauty and you smile to show your appreciation. The sun is behind you and all the sunflowers are smiling at you, radiating positively and optimistically in your face. You are glowing, your face lights up with happiness and cheer.

You then remember a particular time in your life when you felt great pleasure and happiness. Dwelling on this moment brings forward other memories of similar joys, and for a time you were lost in the past. The sound of a bee, buzzing near your ear, brings you back to the present. You begin to contemplate your current circumstances and wonder how you can improve them. You consider the future and all its possibilities and wonder what life has in store for you in a year's time, or three, or five, even ten. But for the moment all you want is to experience the joy of walking among the sunflowers.

With their heads turned to face the sun, they and you are glowing in an orb of GOLDEN YELLOW light, radiating light continuously. They know whichever way they turn, they are filled with this light. It suddenly dawns on you that this is true for you too. Wherever you go, you carry the light with you. You are an instrument of light. This makes you very happy and glad to be alive.

Green Meadow

Picture yourself sitting one afternoon upon a GREEN hill. You are surrounded by other hills, adorned with clusters of trees. The wind gently whispers in your ear and brushes against leaves which shimmer in the clear daylight. The sky is clear, broken by some clouds slowly passing by. You feel the perfect peace and stillness that surrounds you and enjoy the sense of freedom and easiness of the moment. The smooth, rich and vibrant GREEN grass embraces you and seem to touch the very core of your being. You feel hopeful and glad to be alive, thankful for the beauty of life and the simple pleasures it brings. Everywhere you look you see harmony and balance. You feel a deep sense of surety and of protectiveness. No matter what challenges life brings, you will feel safe and secure that everything will be all right.

Turquoise Waterfall

You are on a narrow path on the edge of a rocky mountain and you are following the sounds of gushing water, rumbling over large boulders and trickling through every nook and cranny, as it makes its way down to meet the sea. As you descend, you come across an opening in the side of the mountain, where sunlight streams through, reflecting on to a pool of clear fresh water. A waterfall opposite the opening brings the place alive.

Splashing and cascading folds of effervescent WHITE foam and sparkling drops of water fall like diamonds on to a rippling bed of water. It is a sight you will never forget. You begin to feel replenished and re-energised, even without touching the water or bathing in it.

The temptation is over-powering: you strip off your clothes and walk into the water and feel the silken quality of the TURQUOISE energy at work. Swim over to the edge of the waterfall and let the flow of water cleanse you, feel the pressure of the water drops bounce off your body. Enjoy every second of the natural TURQUOISE colour healing you. Now swim back to your clothes which are resting on the rocks and feel your whole body tingle with energy and vitality. When you are ready, put on your clothes and make your way down to the bottom of the mountain to the sea.

Blue Seas

You are sitting on the deck of a sailing boat far out to sea. It is early in the morning, maybe five or six o'clock and the sky is a perfect pale blue without clouds. It is soft and peaceful. For miles and miles around you there is nothing else but you, your boat, the soft blue sky and the blue velvet sea. In fact, because you are so alone your vision is unobstructed and undisturbed, enabling you to see the horizon's curve.

Where the sky meets the sea, the horizon seems to show itself as a distinct dark blue line, dividing heaven and earth. The sea is quiet and still, and generates feelings of incredible peace and healing. You are alone, but you feel connected and in touch with the whole universe. The only movement is the rippling of the water as the boat gently sails through the morning breeze. You watch, mesmerised, the rippling effect of the water breaking. You are in a state of complete rest and relaxation.

As the sun rises, the sky is filled and bathed in a golden glow of radiant light, which reflects on to the glistening surface of the sea and brings you back.

Violet Mountains

Imagine a wide expanse of land and sky in front of you. It is approximately 8 o'clock one late summer's evening. You are looking out of a very tall building into the distance. In the distance you see a range of PURPLE VIOLET mountains, standing firm and majestically guarding the city. The atmosphere is dull with mist and humidity. To your right PURPLE woods stretch as far as the eye can see. Ribbons of GREY, PURPLE and VIOLET adorn the evening sky, and SILVERY streaks float mysteriously in their shadow. To the left AMETHYST-shadowed rocks adorn the sea-shore and greet the golden YELLOW sands. The air is fresh and crisp, the wind is strong and warns of an impending storm.

As the dim light fades and the clouds draw in, they hang heavy in the sky and the wind strengthens. Suddenly the sounds of thunder breaks and a gentle drizzle of rain begins to fall. Within seconds the drizzle becomes a heavy downpour and everything is washed with rainwater. For some time the rain kept falling, but now it has stopped. The atmosphere is clear, bright and refreshing. Everything has been revitalised, the clouds have dispersed and the light now radiates on all things below. A pleasant aroma drifts your way, and you notice the LILAC wisteria growing up the side of the building.

Magenta Pink Haze

You are taking a leisurely stroll in the countryside one Spring afternoon. You are walking down a leafy country lane with tall grass banks on either side. There is a slight breeze in the air, which you welcome. In the distance you notice a PINK haze of colour and you decide to make your way towards it. As you approach this haze of colour you realise the PINK MAGENTA haze is the blossom from a cherry tree in full bloom. The closer you get to the tree, the more inviting, and the stronger and brighter the colours appear to be. Soft pale PINKS and ROSY PINKS are dusted and fringed with streaks of WHITE, FUSHSIA, CERISE and PINK. The overhanging branches hang heavily with bunches of delicate flowers, filled with the promise of love, gentleness, kindness and compassion, and they sway easily in the fresh, clean air.

Having reached the tree, you stop in amazement and for a moment your breath is taken away. The sight is almost too good for words. As you look up into a soft world of PINK cottonwool surroundings, you imagine yourself like a baby in a heavenly crib. There you stand underneath an umbrella of radiant beauty, as petals softly fall in the breeze, like confetti upon your head and shoulders. Below you the ground is carpeted with PINK, ROSE and MAGENTA petals. For a moment you experience the beauty and glory of the MAGENTA, PINK haze.

Colour Affirmations

Creating a colour affirmation should be based on your needs as revealed by your third colour choice in the Colour Reflection Reading. The affirmation must refer to that particular colour.

An affirmation is a conscious, positive thought that you introduce regularly to your consciousness in order to produce a specific desired result. By constantly repeating this thought or idea you can influence your mind to attract or create what you want. The same process which can be used towards positive results, for good reasons, is also used to enhance negative beliefs about ourselves and others, although this is usually done unconsciously.

There are many different ways to use affirmations in a conscious and positive way. An accepted way is to write down your negative thoughts in a positive form, and we are going to show you how to use this method using the power of colour. Each colour has the potential to strengthen our affirmation through its specific energy, and we will give some examples of how this works. You need to name the colour, relating it to the affirmation you are using with the word 'in', 'through' or 'with'. It will also help to include yourself in the affirming: 'I, Sally . . .' or 'I, Richard . . .'.

Below is a list of words which will help you to transform negative beliefs into positive ideas. Start by focusing on the third colour choice from your CRR, then choose a specific word, or a number of words from the colour affirmation word list. These must be related to your goal and its associated colour as clearly as possible. To be sure the word(s) you choose reflect your third colour choice, refer to the qualities given in the interpretation section in Chapter 1 and the section on enhancing and diminishing colour qualities from Chapter 2. If you do not find the word(s) to describe your negative belief in the word list, then add your new word(s) to the list with their positive counterpart.

Colour Affirmation Word List

RED		ORANGE	
Negative	*Positive*	*Negative*	*Positive*
cold	warm	lifeless	exuberant
feeble	strong	melancholy	fun
angry	patient	depressing	enlivening
exhausted	alive	cowardly	courageous
weak-willed	determined	deliberating	spontaneous
unfriendly	friendly	solitary	sociable
impractical	practical	solemn	humorous
unfeeling	passionate	depleted	vital

RED

Negative	Positive
submissive	assertive
indolent	energetic
following	initiating
apathetic	engaged

ORANGE

Negative	Positive
destructive	constructive
fearful	confident
restrained	impulsive
reluctant	willing

YELLOW

Negative	Positive
irrational	reasonable
illogical	logical
stupid	intelligent
heavy	light
pessimistic	optimistic
inarticulate	articulate
dark	light
malicious	benevolent
vindictive	forgiving
sad	happy
disorderly	orderly
nervous	assured

GREEN

Negative	Positive
imbalanced	balanced
inefficient	efficient
irregular	methodical
unjust	just
unappreciative	appreciative
insincere	sincere
disharmonious	harmonious
threatened	protective
selfish	sharing
trapped	free
insecure	secure
jealous	contented

TURQUOISE

Negative	Positive
dull	sparkling
elderly	youthful
unimaginative	imaginative
disturbed	calm
restrained	transformational
toxic	clean
insensitive	sensitive
unchanging	changing
lowering	elevating
confused	clear
uncertain	evident
unsuccessful	triumphant

BLUE

Negative	Positive
discordant	peaceful
disturbed	tranquil
active	passive
distrusting	faithful
dishonest	honest
unreliable	reliable
isolated	united
escaping	accepting
inflexible	flexible
withdrawn	steadfast
depressed	joyful
intimidating	reassuring

VIOLET		MAGENTA	
Negative	*Positive*	*Negative*	*Positive*
alone	together	unkind	kind
unworthy	valuable	opposed	supportive
undignified	dignified	selfish	considerate
calculating	intuitive	suffering	relief
denying	acknowledging	merciless	compassionate
hidden	revealed	immature	mature
unattractive	beautiful	unloving	loving
humble	proud	artificial	genuine
narrow-minded	open-minded	unhelpful	helpful
vulnerable	impregnable	arrogant	natural
humiliated	admired	small	great
vanity	modesty	stubborn	yielding

How to Construct a Colour Affirmation

From the colours you chose in the Colour Reflection Reading, focus on the third colour, which reflects both our conscious desires for the future and some deeply unconscious needs. To clarify how this works, here is the example of Paul, who came to us for a CRR. His first colour was GREEN, his second YELLOW, his third TURQUOISE, and around these choices we gave him the four basic steps for a colour affirmation.

1. Based on the interpretation of the third colour (TURQUOISE) and what arose from this, we suggested that Paul write down all the negative thoughts and feelings relating to his immediate goals. These could be summed up as basically (a) confusion and (b) uncertainty.

2. To help you find the positive or negative qualities that relate to each colour, use the colour affirmation words listed on p. 154.

3. Now, without thought or delay, write down the opposite, positive qualities. The one which Paul chose were: (a) clarity and (b) certainty.

4. Based on these positive qualities, contruct your own colour affirmation (see pp. 157–159). Paul's looked like this:

'I, Paul, experience greater clarity in my life and am certain of my immediate direction through the colour TURQUOISE.'

5. Now that you have constructed your colour affirmation and you feel satisfied that it feels right to you, write the sentence down and repeat it several times, while visualising the colour.

6. We recommend that you repeat your affirmation for at least five minutes first thing in the morning and last thing at night. You may also want to repeat it at various times during the day. It might be helpful to have your affirmation on a small piece of appropriately coloured card so that you can carry it around with you, or place it somewhere you will see it often.

Some Colour Affirmations

Here are some other colour affirmations which will help to give you an idea of how to construct your own.

Red
'Every day, I, _____, am energised and revitalised by the colour RED.'

'I, _____, am practical and capable of taking responsibility in my life through the power and energy of the colour RED.'

'I, _____, experience through the colour RED, being more assertive than ever before.'

'Through the colour RED, I, _____, feel my body filled with new life and strength.'

Orange
I, _____, experience spontaneity with the colour ORANGE.'

'Through the colour ORANGE, I, _____, am becoming more confident.'

'In ORANGE, I, _____, enjoy socialising and relating to people.'

'Through the colour ORANGE, I, _____, am filled with fun and humour.'

Yellow

'Every day I, _____, am becoming more intelligent and able to articulate myself through the colour YELLOW.'

'I, _____, find it increasingly easy to be optimistic through the colour YELLOW.'

'Every day I, _____, experience my life becoming more orderly and fulfilling through the colour YELLOW.'

'I, _____, am filled with light and happiness through the radiance of the colour YELLOW.'

Green

'Through the colour GREEN, I, _____, easily express my emotions.'

'With the colour GREEN, I, _____, feel secure and protected.'

'I, _____, now recognise my ability to remain centred and balanced at all times with the colour GREEN.'

'Through the colour GREEN, I, _____, am more efficient and methodical in my life.'

Turquoise

'I, _____, experience my body young and healthy through the colour TURQUOISE.'

'The colour TURQUOISE is transformational. I, _____, feel uplifted and elevated by its effects.'

'Through the colour TURQUOISE, I, _____, am becoming more creative and imaginative in my work.'

'Through the colour TURQUOISE I, _____, am becoming more aware of my refreshing nature and the valuable contribution I can offer to others.'

Blue

'Through the colour BLUE, I, _____, am attaining more peace and tranquillity in my life.'

'I, _____, find my strength lies in verbally expressing myself through the colour BLUE.'

'Through the colour BLUE, I, _____, am becoming more honest with myself and other people.'

'Through the colour BLUE, I, _____, find I am supported in being flexible and reliable in life.'

Violet
'In the colour VIOLET I, _____, deserve acknowledgement, recognition and respect from other people.'

I, _____, experience my artistic talents and creativity through the colour VIOLET.'

'Every day I, _____, experience my memory improve with the help of the colour VIOLET.'

'Through the colour VIOLET, I, _____, find spiritual strength in being modest and humble in life.'

Magenta
'I, _____, deserve to receive as well as to give through the colour MAGENTA.'

'Every day I, _____, am becoming more generous and giving in relationships through the colour MAGENTA.'

'Through the colour MAGENTA I, _____, love myself and also allow others love me.'

'I, _____, offer my support and kindness wherever it is needed through the colour MAGENTA.'

The Creative Colour Technique

The Creative Colour Technique was developed from the work of Living Colour. It is an excellent method which works through mental colour projection and the Colour Reflection Reading. Having practised colour breathing, colour visualisation and colour affirmation techniques separately, you may combine them in the same order to make the whole process more focused and powerful. This may seem awkward at first, but it becomes easy with practice. Combining these techniques together works best when the second and third colours are complementary to one another – in other words, when they are in harmony. It is also effective when based on the third colour alone.

Here is a summary of the steps to take.

1. Turn your attention to the colour that came up as your third choice.

2. Start the exercise with a few minutes of normal breathing and relaxation.

3. Begin deep breathing, and start to sense the energy of the third colour.

4. After a few more minutes, introduce the colour visualisation while continuing to breathe deeply and keep focusing on the energy of the colour of your third choice. Do this for ten minutes.

5. Having already chosen and written down your colour affirmation in advance, start to repeat this either silently or aloud as you come to the end of the exercise.

6. Consciously align the rhythm of your breathing with the repetition of your affirmation and relate these to the flow of your visual images, while all the time sensing the quality of the colour energy. Continue for a few minutes and then relax.

The practice time for the combined Creative Colour Technique is about 20 minutes in all.

The Creative Colour Technique works in two distinct stages – internally and externally. The first uses the colour energy of the third colour you chose, through colour breathing, colour visualisation and colour affirmation. The second is to use the colour of your third choice when you see it in your environment. This helps to make your experience more tangible, alive and practical. Use it at your discretion!

Whenever you see the colour on which your affirmation is based in the environment around you, you will be reminded of the essence of the affirmation, and this will encourage you to repeat it consciously to yourself. Practise regularly and there will come a time when you no longer need to say the words: the message will be immediately received. By regularly noticing the colour alone, and acknowledging the message which it has for you, the positive thought will become imprinted in your mind, and your goal will be closer to reality. Working with affirmations in this way helps you to acknowledge your own needs and what needs to be done about them, and also develops your awareness of colour.

Think how many times you can introduce positive healing and creative energy into your life through colour. For instance, a person who chooses blue as their third colour can be reminded of their affirmation every time they encounter a blue flower, item of clothing, picture, or object. Anything which is blue can act as a reminder. So awaken yourself to your aims and use the creative power of colour to achieve them.

chapter 8

■ ◆ ▲ ● ▼ ◆ ◆

COLOUR THERAPY

Before turning directly to colour therapy and how we use it, it would be helpful to glance briefly at some of the physical aspects of light and its effect both on humans and plants.

The Effects of Light and Colour

The source of all light is the sun. Light from the sun is filled with electromagnetic energy, travelling at the speed of light (186,000 miles per second) but on different frequencies, and with different wavelengths. As the nearest star to our planet Earth, it would seem its chief function is to supply us with enormous amounts of electro-magnetic energy which sustains and nourishes all living organisms – plant, animal and human life. In plants the energy from natural daylight is captured by chlorophyll (the GREEN pigments that gives most plants their colour) and is used to make up complex organic molecules within the plant cells. This process is commonly known as photosynthesis and emphasises the close links between light and life, since directly or indirectly it feeds us all. For example, without light plants turn WHITISH or YELLOW in colour and usually have underdeveloped leaves as a result of chlorophyll deficiency.

In 1895 C. Flammarion discovered that RED light offered the best effects for the growth of plants. He noted that plants under the effects of RED and ORANGE light seemed to produce taller plants with thinner leaves than those grown under BLUE light, which causes them to grow relatively weak and underdeveloped in comparison.

Just as insufficient light causes deficiencies in plants and humans, so too the over-exposure of intense light upon plants can cause adverse affects. The long wavelengths of infrared and the short wavelengths of ultraviolet have both been found to be detrimental to, and will eventually destroy, plant life. Yet these same rays have been accepted to be of therapeutic value to human beings. Why should these rays have such opposite effects on plants and humans? More research needs to be undertaken if we are to realise the valuable role colour can play in the future of medicine as a more accepted form of therapy.

One thing is certain, the human body does respond to light. Infrared light produces heat within the body which is used for the treatment of neuralgia. Ultraviolet light also helps to keep the skin healthy and is recognised for the vital production of vitamin D in the body, and the destruction of germs. Too much exposure to ultraviolet light causes malignant skin tumours at worst and to a lesser degree encourages wrinkles and tends to quicken the ageing process.

How We See Colour and Light

The way human beings see the world is partly determined by the physical workings and mechanics of how the eye works, and the range of colours we can see is partly dependent on the chemical properties of certain pigments in the retina.

Within the retina there are special light receptor cells called the rods and the cones, named after their shapes. It is these cells which begin the process of transforming the patterns we experience into electrical brain patterns. The rods regulate the amount of light we see, i.e. BLACK and WHITE. These cells are sensitive to low levels of light and are used for night vision. The cones regulate the quality of light received and this enables us to see colour. The cones in general can form much sharper images than that of the rods, partly because they absorb greater intensities of light generally. It is known that there are three types of cones, those sensitive primarily to RED, to BLUE and GREEN. All the colours we perceive through vision are formed from these three primaries. When the pulsations of electrical impulses are received by the brain the brain adds its judgement and perception to what it receives and 'sees'.

The light that passes through the eyes via the retina continues its journey along the route to the brain and the hypothalamus. The hypothalamus is a structure deep within the brain which controls the pineal and pituitary glands, which in turn stimulates and regulates hormonal and neurochemical functions. The hypothalamus is concerned with the vital functions of the body and its integrity is essential for life. It is part of a system that controls the physiological expressions of our emotions. The pineal and the pituitary glands are both susceptible to light. The pituitary is known as the 'master' gland of the other endocrine glands which comprise part of the autonomic nervous system. This controls the involuntary functions such as heartbeat, circulation and pupil movements of the eye, as well as regulating our mood towards others.

Experiments from the 1950s to 1970s using bedside lights to shorten and regularise menstrual cycles suggest that light may be used to treat infertility, aid in contraception and help in other endocrine disorders.

Light and colour therefore seem to have 'nutritional' value, providing us with vital elements to sustain and nourish our bodies, and they have the potential to effect subtle chemical changes within our body to help the healing processes of certain diseases.

Light Is Not Just for Seeing

Light enters the body through two channels, the eyes and skin. The action of light on the skin produces melanin, storing and replenishing the body's supply of vitamin D. The vitamin D passes into the bloodstream and makes its way to the kidneys and liver, where it plays a vital role in allowing absorption of calcium from the diet, which is then used to repair bones and teeth.

An ailment known as Seasonal Affective Disorder (SAD for short), affects millions of people all over the world who suffer from depression and social withdrawal, fatigue, oversleeping, reduced sexual drive, lack of concentration, general diminished use of mental activity, headaches and often cravings for carbohydrates. It results from a deficiency of sunlight and has been described as the 'Winter Blues', as many sufferers experience the symptoms between mid-autumn and spring.

If it's winter-time and you've been feeling depressed, lethargic and disinterested in social activity, maybe you are experiencing some of the effects of this syndrome. Try spending more of your time outdoors, and taking daily walks or outdoor exercises like jogging or running. Try choosing a desk near a window to work, or set up a study in the sunniest room of the house. Choose a home with lots of windows, keep the hedges trimmed low and the windows unshaded. If you suffer acutely from SAD, and if you can possibly afford it, try taking a winter holiday in a sunny climate.

As an alternative, various types of instruments and bulbs which artificially simulate natural light have been designed to treat the disorder successfully. These instruments use fluorescent tubes which reflect a balanced spectrum of natural light and are known as full spectrum light. The effects of using these instruments seem to compensate for the shortages of our exposure to light from the sun. Patients sit for approximately six hours a day in front of special light-boxes which emit light of extremely high intensities to help ease their complaints.

One interesting case reported in a British national newspaper in 1986 referred to a woman writer in her early thirties with two small children, who suffered from the usual symptoms of SAD. She sat in front of lights which simulated natural light, five times as bright as normal indoor lighting, for several hours in the mornings and in the evenings. Her reaction was dramatic. She reported, 'After a few days I felt re-energised and while under the lights finished an article I had previously been unable to start. I even felt repelled by a huge chocolate gateau on the cover of a gourmet magazine. The change was so definite I felt as if someone had thrown a chemical switch in my body.'

Ordinary fluorescent lighting comes in basically two types: warm (RED) biased and cool (BLUE) biased. The warm types give out a YELLOWISH light, and the cool types a BLUE/WHITE light. In recent years fluorescent lighting has been linked with various health disorders, especially where people are exposed to it over long periods. Apart from the incorrect colour balance and the flickering effect, the sheer volume of artificial light to which it exposes us can promote stress, headaches, tiredness, irritability, an inability to concentrate, and nausea. Their inventor never intended them to be used on the scale they are today. In fact he judged them unsafe for use over long periods. They spread largely because of the need for cheap electricity during the last world war.

An improvement on the use of the ordinary household bulb is the development of the daylight bulb, which is supposed to simulate natural light in artificial form. Its natural BLUE-coloured glass filters the excess of RED light characteristic of normal household bulbs and has been reported to improve alertness and concentration, reduce eyestrain and to aid against stress, headaches and depression. People experience this type of lighting as being softer and more restful on the eyes. It also seems to be of great benefit to plants as well as to humans.

Daylight Bulbs can be obtained through Living Colour. For details see p. 182.

Coloured Light

To subject yourself directly to intense coloured light is to enter the realm of colour therapy and is not recommended without supervision from a skilled practitioner. Coloured light is one of the most powerful ways of using colour as it works on the whole body through the nervous system. Living Colour employs particular colours and varying intensities in relation to specific physical and emotional problems to compensate for deficiencies of colour energy in the system. We consider the specific intensity level, duration of exposure and so on, in order to treat a person for their individual imbalance. The wrong use of coloured lights can create adverse effects within us. For example, exposure to a random selection of colours from the spectrum usually leaves us feeling dizzy, nauseous and strained. So coloured lights must be used with caution.

On major research project into the effects of colour and light upon humans was undertaken by Robert Gerard, an American scientist. In 1932 he experimented on prisoners using coloured lights. First he exposed them to RED light and found they became restless, agitated and even aggressive in behaviour. RED, he documented in his report, created feelings of anxiety and tended to stimulate the heartbeat and respiration rate as well as muscular activity. Prisoners generally experienced an increase in physiological and mental activity. BLUE on the other hand created calming and tranquillising effects. BLUE had the reverse effects to those of RED, creating feelings of sedation and relaxation. Physiologically the blood pressure was decreased, and respiratory and muscular activity were reduced compared with using RED.

In our work the use of colour illumination has been used to treat constipation, psoriasis, stomach ulcers, prostate problems, low/high blood pressure, various eye problems, breathing difficulties, bowel problems, stress, anaemia, throat conditions etc. on the physiological side. Problems related to lack of confidence, relationship difficulties, sexual problems and various kinds of phobias on the psychological side have also been treated.

But to use coloured lights safely and effectively in terms of treating a physical or psychological problem, it is essential to be familiar with the principles of colour therapy, for which you would need to undertake a course such as the ones we teach at Living Colour (see p. 182).

What Is Colour Therapy?

Colour therapy is the art of re-introducing different spectral hues into the human organism, in order to promote health, balance and general well-being. Colour vibration is absorbed through the subtle fields of energy around the human body (i.e. the aura). These vibrations are also absorbed through the eyes and skin, as well as the power centres (i.e. the chakras) which are associated with the endocrine system. The regulation of colour entering and leaving these systems enables physical, emotional and mental restoration, rebuilding and revitalising every organ in the body and their etheric counterpart. The effects of colour therapy on the human system help to align the body, mind and emotions. This alignment through the power of colour promotes personal growth and spiritual development.

The Principles of Colour Therapy Treatment

The principles of colour therapy seem, at first, to be simple. That is, most people consider once they have learnt the meanings of each colour, positive and negative, and feel able to associate these qualities with the specific chakra absorbing those qualities, they can then practise colour therapy. This could not be further from the truth. Having said this, it *is* necessary to become really familiar with each colour. In other words, you do need to know the action of each colour physically, emotionally and mentally. This helps to lay one of the basic foundations which will serve you in any future work you do with colour. But this knowledge is not enough to be used on its own as a form of healing or from which to administer colour. Nor should it be the basis to recommend colour for someone else. Every person must be seen as an individual and when it comes to advising or administering colour therapy, they must be treated as an individual. Since every person's needs are different, the recommendations and administrations of colour applying to their needs must be personal to them.

How Can Colour Therapy Be Applied?

Probably the most obvious way of receiving the complete range of colours from the spectrum is to expose yourself to natural sunlight, as the ancient Greeks and Egyptians used to do. Unfortunately it is not always possible to receive the therapeutic rays from the sun whenever we want or indeed whenever we need them, and therefore colour therapy instruments have been created to serve this purpose. Such instruments can also isolate specific colour rays from within the spectrum and can project on to the body generally, or even on to a particular part of the body as required.

Colour therapy can be applied to the body physically by exposing it to artificial coloured lights which are emitted from specially designed colour therapy instruments. One such instrument is the Colour Light Crystal Unit produced by Living Colour. This is a portable instrument measuring 20 in high, 20 in wide and 12 in deep, which is capable of using different coloured filters, both stained-glass and the plastic cinemoid filters commonly used in theatres. It is also able to project coloured light through a large crystal. The instrument provides a variable light intensity option and is operated via a compact control box.

Other forms of applying colour therapy are through mental projection, meditation and techniques of suggestion, such as visualisation and affirmation. These methods of using colour can be seen as harnessing our inherent and creative healing abilities, fundamentally tapping into our own inner light and the surrounding universal energies.

Each of us is subjected to a constant, inexhaustible source of energy, received from the Earth and the cosmos. As conscious, intelligent human beings we can learn to use this energy for positive use, through regular practice of quiet meditational exercises. We will soon realise that the power to effect healing actually lies within us and more often than not this power tends to lie dormant. This is usually because we tend to look for solutions and answers to our problems outside of ourselves rather than looking within. We fail to recognise the power of healing and most of us are too busy undermining our own strength and inherent abilities. To put this energy and power to constructive use implies we have the potential to alleviate ill-health and disease to a large degree, when it occurs, and also to use it as a form of preventative therapy. In the previous chapter we looked at some of the principles of the above techniques which deal with inner light and self-healing.

This book essentially focuses around the Colour Reflection Reading process and thereby places a great deal of attention upon how colour affects our emotions. In 1987 Living Colour adopted the phrase 'colour counselling' to describe the process of giving a CRR and pursuing in-depth counselling based on the main issues that arise during the interpretation. Colour counselling focuses on these areas separately while still taking into account the overall state of the patient. The colour counsellor aims to support and encourage the patient by enabling them to come to terms with unresolved areas or issues in their life by synthesising counselling skills with colour psychology and colour awareness.

There are several other ways of applying colour therapy, some of which are not mentioned in this book. These include exercise, foods, gems and crystals. These can also be considered as everyday, practical forms of bringing more colour into your life.

The Living Colour Approach

When a client comes to Living Colour for a Colour Reflection Reading, they are asked to complete a simple form giving their basic details and their colour preferences. As part of this session, colour advice may be included (where appropriate) and they will receive a colour therapy treatment based on the main colour recommended in the Reading. This session usually lasts for an hour and a half.

There are two possible ways you can pursue your interest:

1. A course of Colour Reflection Readings given at three monthly intervals for a period of approximately 12 months. These sessions check and monitor how you are doing, having now had the opportunity to put the advice from the previous session into practice.

2. A course of colour therapy treatment.

A Course of Living Colour Therapy Sessions

Here a patient comes for monthly colour therapy sessions. A full course lasts from nine to 12 months. At the 'orientation' session the client completes an application form, giving details of their general state of health, their current and previous medical history, and their likes and dislikes for particular colours. Colour counselling follows in order to prepare the patient for the course of colour–light treatment.

To receive colour–light treatment, a colour spine chart has to be drawn up. To make a colour spine chart, the completed application form is placed underneath the spine chart. This chart is then used by the colour therapist to dowse and 'pick up' any colour imbalances or disharmonies that may exist.

The chart itself is a printed copy of the spinal column where each vertebrae is associated with a particular colour. Since the spine is connected through the nervous system to all parts of the body, each vertebra is associated with a particular organ. The process of picking up imbalanced sensations involves the colour therapist scanning each vertebra, while keeping the image of the patient in their mind.

Imbalances can be experienced as tingling, pricking, hot or cold sensations which indicate where the imbalance exists and which colour is required to balance it. This method of dowsing, usually using the middle finger, is one learnt in the advance stages of practising colour therapy and requires concentration, acute stillness and observation. These colour spine charts also indicate the main colour needed for treatment and any subsequent follow-up sessions where colour–light treatment is administered. In the case where a client cannot attend colour–light treatment sessions, the application form is used by the colour therapist as the basis on which to project mentally colour therapy and send absent healing.

A case history

A couple of years ago Sally came to the Living Colour Centre to receive colour therapy treatment for the first time. She had discovered that a hard rounded mass of tissue (about 1½ inches in size) had developed on the outer side of her right breast. This cyst was unsightly and causing her some concern. Her specialist had recommended that the cyst be surgically removed in case a tumour might develop. She was glad to know she did not have cancer, but was unhappy with the recommended solution to her problem, i.e. surgery. It was at this point that she came to see us. She wanted to know if colour therapy could help her to remove the cyst. Of course no guarantee could be given, but we said that we'd see what we could do.

Our patient chose MAGENTA for her first colour from the Colour Reflection Reading, GREEN for her second and BLUE for her third. These colours seemed exactly to reflect her personality, personal circumstances and needs.

During her colour therapy treatment sessions which lasted for nine months, she was able to reduce the hardened mass of tissue completely. She experienced MAGENTA as the main colour for therapy, which was of course complemented with GREEN. Only on one occasion did she actually receive GREEN as the main colour for therapy. She was also given colour breathing, colour visualisation and colour affirmation exercises to do, at least twice a day, morning and night. She was asked to incorporate the colours she needed in her clothes and in her environment. By using the Creative Colour Technique as well, she became increasingly conscious of colour in her life and she was able to improve her condition steadily over a nine-month period, which meant that she was also working on a preventative level.

After three months she had a hospital check-up, and although at this stage the cyst had not disappeared, it had reduced to almost half its original size. The specialist and hospital staff couldn't understand it! After nine months she visited the hospital again, to confirm that her cyst had completely disappeared. It had. Her specialist told her that he did not need to see her again unless the cyst should reappear. To this day she has not had the need to go back.

For Sally, as with all the clients we have treated, the healing goes beyond the symptoms alone. At the end of her course of therapy, Sally understood more about herself and had a geater awareness of what had led to this problem happening in her life and the contributory factors that supported it. She came to terms with her problem and its impact. As a result she gained some major insights into her personality and understood how she could help prevent imbalances of this kind from repeating themselves in the future. Overall, she felt a more balanced and powerful individual. She realised that she was more able to deal with stressful situations and was a happier person altogether. She recognised that her illness had been the catalyst in opening up a whole new perception of herself.

CONCLUSION

Throughout this book we have described some of the fundamental principles of colour therapy and how they can be used effectively and practically to bring more colour into your life. We have shared the Colour Reflection Reading, a useful tool through which most of the other techniques described can be worked.

Essentially our aim has been to encourage greater self-awareness and consciousness, by increasing your awareness of your own needs through the medium of colour. If you lack colour in your life, you may be described as being 'colourless', or 'wanting in character'. Bringing more colour into your lives adds character and vitality to your personality.

The Colour Reflection Reading helps you to create a more complete picture of who you really are. People have described it as being like looking into a mirror and seeing their true reflection in colour. We hope that you too will have begun a process of seeing yourself in a different light and that this will bring about positive and worthwhile changes in your life.

appendix

■ ◆ ▲ ● ▼ ◆ ◆

LIVING COLOUR LOGO

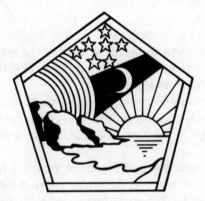

You may be interested in the Living Colour Logo, which appears above and on the cover. It was developed from a painting called *Manifestation*, designed by myself in 1983 and submitted as part of my final dissertation when I completed my colour training. This picture is symbolic and embodies the essence of the Living Colour philosophy about personal growth and human consciousness.

There are basically five main stages of manifestations which all living things must pass through from the spirit world into the gross material world. Each state is one of evolution or consciousness.

As a 'True Self' we consciously choose to descend from the higher realms into lower, physical ones. It is in the spiritual realms we set forth the idea to incarnate as a human being and begin the process of manifestation and begin our descent. In this way we choose our parents, the particular environment and background necessary to influence and support our individual required experiences on Earth.

The five stages of manifestation are: darkness, light, colour, sound and form.

Darkness   Seen in the logo as the black shaft of light coming down from the ocean of universal energy. Darkness, an energy in its own right, acts as the point from which its opposite light can spring forth. Darkness, the unknown, seen as the mysterious dimensions of life, not yet physical, but filled with spirituality. Out of the darkness came light.

Light   The reflector or mirror image of our inner and true spiritual essence. In the logo this is seen as the sun, radiating light and life on all things. Light gives birth to all biological forms, plants, animals, humans even minerals. It is the light within us which constantly radiates and expresses pure love. This being the purpose of our descent – to learn to love.

When the extreme forces of the universe, darkness and light, meet and interact, and merge together, colour springs forth. In nature we see this in the birth of a rainbow in the sky.

Colour   Seen in the logo as the rainbow, radiating from out of the heavens on to the Earth. It is the bridge between the spiritual and the physical worlds. When darkness and light meet, colour is created. Colour becomes a natural balancing energy force which can act as a powerful medium for healing purposes. It aids our development, enabling us to shape our emotional and psychic bodies, so that when we manifest physically, we are more able to express our essence. At this stage we are only light beings, we have not yet manifested physically. We must first evolve through each of the eight colours of the spectrum from RED through to MAGENTA in order to move into the next stage of development, which is sound.

Sound   When we descend through the stages of colour, the light vibrations become gradually more dense. When colour ceases to be colour and becomes sound instead, it passes through the atmosphere as inaudible sound, then as the vibrations become slower and more dense, sound becomes audible and it becomes 'frozen sound'. In the logo, sound is depicted as swirls of energy moving with the forces of the universe.

Form Out of 'frozen sound' comes solidity and physical matter. 'Frozen sound' becomes more and more durable until it eventually manifests into a visible, tangible and permanent substance. Form is then manifested for the first time and takes on the idea of something solid. In the logo this is seen in the manifestation of the landscape of the Earth.

The shape in which these scenes are all contained is the pentagram. The pentagram has five sides, each side represents one stage of manifestation. The pentagram is also the symbol for universal wholeness, unity and love. Each side of the pentagram has an associated colour. (Top left side) GREEN; (top right side) MAGENTA; (left side) YELLOW; (right side) BLUE; and (bottom side) RED. These colours connect with five elements. RED with Fire, YELLOW with Air, GREEN with Earth, BLUE, with Water and MAGENTA with Ether.

Dorothy Sun

BIBLIOGRAPHY

Anderson, Jan (1981), *Colour Revolution*, Anderson Press.
Babbit, Edwin (1967, 2nd edition), *The Principles of Light and Colour*, Citadel Press.
Birren, Faber (1980), *Colour*, Marshall Editions.
Birren, Faber (1950), *Colour Psychology and Colour Therapy*, Citadel Press.
Birren, Faber (1970), *Colour and the Human Response*, Van Nostrand Reinhold.
Clark, Linda (1975), *The Ancient Art of Colour Therapy*, Pocket Books.
Gawain, Shakti (1979), *Creative Visualization*, Pantone New Age Books.
Hunt, Roland (1941), *Lighting – Therapy and Colour Harmony*, C. M. Daniel.
Gimbel, Theo (1980), *Healing through Colour*, C. M. Daniel.
Jackson, Carole (1983), *Colour Me Beautiful*, Piatkus Books.
Karagulla, Dr Shafica and Dora van Gelder Kunz (1989), *The Chakras and the Human Energy Fields*, The Theosophical Publishing House.
Lüscher, Dr Max (1987), *The Lüscher Colour Test*, Pan Books.
Ray, Sondra (1980), *Loving Relationships*, Celestial Press.
Rossotti, Hazel (1983), *Colour*, Pelican Books.
Tibbs, Hardwin (1981), *The Future of Light*, Watkins.
Wilson, Annie and Lillia Bek (1981), *What Colour Are You?*, Turnstone Press.
Wood, Betty (1984), *The Healing Power of Colour*, Aquarian Press.

INDEX

Page numbers in *italic* refer to the illustrations

A NOTE ON SUN YAT SEN

In China all people with the same surname are said to be related. If this is true then my ancestors ruled the largest and most powerful of the Three Kingdoms in China (222–280 AD). Its capital was situated in Nanking which is also where my family's ancestral temple is located. It is here, where my great-great grand uncle's mausoleum is situated. Sun Yat-Sen (1866–1925) was born in Kwantung province and received his medical training in Hong Kong. When he graduated in 1892 he changed his first name from Tai-cheong to Yat-Sen which means 'unconventional or free spirit'. His outlook was modern which reflected his answer to China's plight – to establish a democratic republic.

Dr Sun Yat-Sen was responsible for instigating the downfall of the last dynasty in China – the Ching Dynasty – after 11 unsuccessful attempts to overthrow them. During his attempts to make China a democratic republic, his life was constantly under threat. Now known as the 'father of modern China', he became the first President of the Republic of China in 1911.

At the first pergola of his impressive mausoleum the words 'Universal Love' are inscribed. These words reflect his ideological beliefs. I feel he was a very special individual, one who saw and responded deeply to the plight of his people. I feel very humble and proud to be related to him. Sun Yat-Sen dedicated his life to help bring about the restoration and the dignity of the Chinese people. In my own way as a teacher and therapist, working to educate, uplift and heal the human spirit, I hope to carry on in the same tradition. In my heart, I truly believe we are kindred spirits and his presence and memory is close to me and lives on as a beacon to China's future.

Howard Sun

FURTHER INFORMATION ABOUT LIVING COLOUR

For more information about Living Colour please write to us, stating your area of interest, and enclose a stamped addressed envelope:

Living Colour
33 Lancaster Grove
Hampstead
London NW3 4EX

Educational
We have a range of courses to support you as you develop your understanding of Colour Therapy. Courses start with the 'Colour Your Life' four-day programme.

Therapeutic
One-to-one treatments are available. They take many forms and always start with a Colour Reflection Reading.

Creative
We supply a small range of products including a set of long-life Colour Reflection Reading cards, Colour Analysis Wallets, Daylight Bulbs, Colour Crystal Light Units and pens.

If you would like to join the Living Colour Association please specify this in your letter.

To receive our Programme Information Pack with full details on how to become a Colour Counsellor or a Colour Therapist, plus information on *all* our services and products, send a cheque for £2.00 (made out to **Living Colour**) to the above address.

Piatkus Books

If you are interested in recovery, health and personal growth, you may like to read other titles published by Piatkus.

RECOVERY

Adult Children of Divorce: *How to achieve happier relationships* Dr Edward W Beal and Gloria Hochman (Foreword by Zelda West-Meads of *RELATE*)

At My Father's Wedding: *Reclaiming our true masculinity* John Lee

Children of Alcoholics: *How a parent's drinking can affect your life*   David Stafford

The Chosen Child Syndrome: *What to do when a parent's love rules your life*   Dr Patricia Love and Jo Robinson

Codependents' Guide to the Twelve Steps: *How to understand and follow a recovery programme*   Melody Beattie

Codependency: *How to break free and live your own life* David Stafford and Liz Hodgkinson

Don't Call it Love: *Recovery from sexual addiction* Dr Patrick Carnes

Homecoming: *Reclaiming and championing your inner child* John Bradshaw

Obsessive Love: *How to free your emotions and live again* Liz Hodgkinson

HEALTH

Acupressure: *How to cure common ailments the natural way* Michael Reed Gach

The Alexander Technique: *How it can help you*   Liz Hodgkinson

Aromatherapy: *The encyclopedia of plants and oils and how they can help you*   Danièle Ryman

Arthritis Relief at Your Fingertips: *How to use acupressure massage to ease your aches and pains*   Michael Reed Gach

The Encyclopedia of Alternative Health Care: *The guide to choices in healing*   Kristin Olsen

Herbal Remedies: *The complete guide to natural healing*   Jill Nice

Hypnosis Regression Therapy: *How reliving early experiences can improve your life*   Ursula Markham

Increase Your Energy: *Regain your zest for life the natural way* Louis Proto

Infertility: *Modern treatments and the issues they raise*
Maggie Jones
Nervous Breakdown: *What is it? What causes it? Who will help?*
Jenny Cozens
The Reflexology Handbook: *A complete guide*
Laura Norman and Thomas Cowan
Self-Healing: *How to use your mind to heal your body*
Louis Proto
The Shiatsu Workbook: *A beginners' guide*   Nigel Dawes
Spiritual Healing: *All you need to know*   Liz Hodgkinson
Super Health: *How to control your body's natural defences*
Christian Godefroy
Super Massage: *Simple techniques for instant relaxation*
Gordon Inkeles
Women's Cancers: *The treatment options*   Donna Dawson

PERSONAL GROWTH

Colour Your Life: *Discover your true personality through colour*
Howard and Dorothy Sun
Dare to Connect: *How to create confidence, trust and loving
relationships*   Susan Jeffers
Fire in the Belly: *On being a man*   Sam Keen
Living Magically: *A new vision of reality*   Gill Edwards
The Passion Paradox: *What to do when one person loves more than the
other*   Dr Dean C Delis with Cassandra Phillips
Protect Yourself: *How to be safe on the streets, in the home, at work,
when travelling*   Jessica Davies
The Power of Gems and Crystals: *How they can transform your
life*   Soozi Holbeche
The Right to be Yourself: *How to be assertive and make changes in your
life*   Tobe Aleksander

For a free brochure with further information on our range of titles,
please write to:

Piatkus Books,
Freepost 7 (WD 4505),
London W1E 4EZ